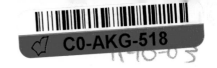

RESEARCH AND PERSPECTIVES IN ALZHEIMER'S DISEASE
Fondation Ipsen

Springer

Berlin
Heidelberg
New York
Hong Kong
London
Milan
Paris
Tokyo

D. J. Selkoe   Y. Christen (Eds.)

Immunization Against Alzheimer's Disease and Other Neurodegenerative Disorders

With 39 Figures and 5 Tables

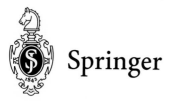

Springer

Selkoe, Dennis J., MD
Center for Neurologic Diseases
Harvard Medical School
and Brigham and Women's Hospital
77 Avenue Louis Pasteur, HIM 730
Boston, MA 02115
USA
e-mail: dselkoe@rics.bwh.harvard.edu

Christen, Yves, Ph.D.
Fondation IPSEN
Pour la Recherche Thérapeutique
24, rue Erlanger
75781 Paris Cedex 16
France
e-mail:
yves.christen@beaufour-ipsen.com

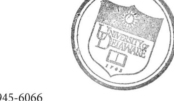

ISSN 0945-6066
ISBN 3-540-00707-5 Springer-Verlag Berlin Heidelberg New York

Cataloging-in-Publication Data applied for
Bibliographic information published by Die Deutsche Bibliothek
Die Deutsche Bibliothek lists this publication in the Deutsche Nationalbibliografie;
detailed bibliographic data is available in the Internet at <http://dnb.ddb.de>.

Springer-Verlag a member of BertelsmannSpringer
Science + Business Media GmbH

http://www.springer.de

© Springer-Verlag Berlin Heidelberg 2003
Printed in Germany

Production: PRO EDIT GmbH, 69126 Heidelberg, Germany
Cover design: design & production, 69121 Heidelberg, Germany
Typesetting and Repro: AM-productions GmbH, 69168 Wiesloch, Germany
Printed on acid-free paper   27/10914250Re – 5 4 3 2 1 0

Preface

The July 1999 publication in *Nature* (Schenk et al. 1999) about the promising effects in mice of immunization by β-amyloid (Aβ) stimulated substantial research efforts and high hopes. In retrospect, this study appears simultaneously logical, consistent as it is with the amyloid theory central today in the field of Alzheimer's disease (AD) studies, and paradoxical, because it involved using the toxic substance itself for a treatment benefit. It has been confirmed and extended by several others (Janus et al. 2000, Morgan et al. 2000, Schenk 2002). Together they suggest that such a "vaccination" can clean the brain of amyloid deposits and favorably modify the animal's behavior. The research thus begun opens up multiple perspectives for experimentation and for treatment. Clinical trials with Aβ42 (under the name AN 1792) began: the phase I studies were encouraging, but the phase II trial, with 375 patients, had to be stopped in January 2002 because of serious side effects (17 cases of meningoencephalitis), that is, only two months before the XVIII° Medical Research Colloquium devoted by the Fondation Ipsen to AD. This book constitutes the proceedings of that meeting, which took place in Paris on 13 March 2002.

The meeting's aim was not limited to the therapeutic prospects for these studies. Most of the specialists present thought that the failure of this first treatment attempt represented not the end of this research pathway but, more probably, in the words of one of the participants, "the end of the beginning" (Schenk 2002). Other possibilities are emerging, such as other immunization routes (nasal, in particular; Weiner et al. 2000), the use of different peptides, or passive immunization directly with the antibody rather than the peptide (Bard et al. 2000; Backsai et al. 2001).

Moreover, many questions arise – about the possibility of immunization against a protein native to the organism, the specific type of immune reactions associated with immunization against Aβ, and immune reactions in elderly subjects. Other studies lead us to wonder about whether the vaccine has necessarily to access to the brain, insofar as there seems to be a dynamic equilibrium between the Aβ of the central nervous system and plasma Aβ: anti-Aβ antibodies may be able to act as a "peripheral sink" and alter this equilibrium (DeMattos et al. 2001).

On the other hand, thanks to the work on immunization against AD, unpredicted discoveries have been made. For example, works using multiphoton microscopy have shown that, in addition to its preventive effect, immunotherapy can clear the existing senile plaques in the brain (Backsai et al. 2001).

The recent analysis of human neuropathology after immunization with AN-1792 Auggest that the immune response generated against Aβ elicited clearance of Aβ plaques in the first patient studied (Nicoll et al. 2003).

It will be especially interesting to see whether the attenuation of the amyloid pathology is accompanied by clinical improvement, and if so, how much. What we can expect from this work is that it will provide clinical confirmation of the validity of the amyloid theory, today supported by substantial theoretical and experimental arguments but not yet demonstrated in humans (Hardy and Selkoe 2002).

Finally, if its medical value is confirmed, immunization may be a therapeutic approach for many neurodegenerative diseases. These seem to involve the aggregation of a particular peptide in the brain – Aβ for AD, α-synuctein for Parkinson's disease and Lewy body dementia, tau in diverse frontal lobe dementias (but also in AD), the PrP^{sc} protein in prion diseases, etc. Immunization trials may therefore be useful in several diseases.

This research therefore opens up numerous prospects and raises as many questions. These justify its choice as the theme in the series of Medical Research Colloquia sponsored by the Fondation Ipsen. It goes without saying that the organizers' and editors' objective for this book is not to arouse false hopes for a therapeutic project that must still be proven but to discuss the available information and the questions it raises.

April 2003   *Yves Christen*

Acknowledgments

We would like to thank the various people who helped in organizing this colloquium, in particular Jacqueline Mervaillie, as well as MaryLynn Gage for her editorial assistance.

References

Backsai B, Kajdasz S, Christie R, Carter C, Games D, Seubert P, Schenk D, Hyman B (2001) Imaging of amyloid β deposits in brains of living mice permits direct observation of clearance of plaques with immunotherapy. Nature Med 7:369–372.

Bard F, Cannon C, Barbour R, Burke R-L, Games D, Grajeda H, Guido T, Hu K, Huang J, Johnson-Wood K, Khan K, Kholodenko D, Lee M, Lieberburg 1, Motter R, Nguyen M, Soriano F, Vasquez N, Weiss K, Welch B, Seubert P, Schenk D, Yednock T (2000) Peripherally administered autoantibodies against amyloid β-peptide enter the central nervous system and reduce pathology in a mouse model of Alzheimer disease. Nature Med 6:916–919.

DeMattos RB, Bales KR, Cummins DJ, Dodart J-C, Paul SM, Holtzman DM (2001) Peripheral anti-Aβ antibody alters CNS and plasma Aβ clearance and decreases brain Aβ burden in a mouse model of Alzheimer's disease. Proc Natl Acad Sci USA 98:8850–8855.

Hardy J, Selkoe D (2002) The amyloid hypothesis of Alzheimer's disease: progress and problems on the road to therapeutics. Science 297:353–356.

Janus C, Pearson J, McLaurin J, Mathews PM, Jiang Y, Schmidt SD, Chishti MA, Horne P, Heslin D, French J, Mount HTJ, Nixon RA, Mercken M, Bergeron C, Fraser PE, St. George-Hyslop P,

Westaway (2000) Aβ peptide immunization reduces behavioural impairment and plaques in a model of Alzheimer's disease. Nature 408:979–982.

Morgan D, Diamond DM, Gottschall PE, Ugen KE, Dickey C, Hardy J, Duff K, Jantzen P, Dicarlo G, Wilcock D, Connor K, Hatcher J, Hope C, Gordon M, Arendash GW (2000) Aβ peptide vaccination prevents memory loss in an animal model of Alzheimer's disease. Nature 408:982–985.

Nicoll JA, Wilkinson D, Holmes C, Steart P, Markham H, Weller RO (2003) Neuropathology of human Alzheimer disease after immunization with amyloid-beta peptide: a case report. Nature Med 9:448–452.

Schenk D (2002) Amyloid-β immunotheray for Alzheimer's disease: the end of the beginning. Nature Rev Neurosci 3:824–828.

Schenk D, Barbour R, Dunn W, Gordon G, Grajeda H, Guido T, Hu K, Huang J, Johnson-Wood K, Khan K, Kholodenko D, Lee M, Liao Z, Lieberburg 1, Motter R, Mutter L, Soriano F, Shopp G, Vasquez N, Vandevert C, Walker S, Wogulis M, Yednock T, Games D, Seubert P (1999) Immunization with amyloid-β attenuates Alzheimer-disease-like pathology in the PDAPP mouse. Nature 400:173–177

Weiner HL, Lemere CA, Maron R, Spooner ET, Grenfell TJ, Mori C, Issazadeh S, Hancock WW, Selkoe DJ (2000) Nasal administration of amyloid-beta peptide decreases cerebral amyloid burden in a mouse model of Alzheimer's disease. Ann Neurol 48:567–579.

Contents

List of Contributors

Bacskai, B.J.
Massachusetts General Hospital/Harvard Medical School,
Department of Neurology, 114, 16th Street (CAGN 2009), Charlestown,
MA 02129, USA, e-mail Bacskai@helix.mgh.harvard.edu

Bai, Y.
Dept. of Medical Microbiology and Immunology,
University of South Florida College of Medicine,
MDC 10, 12901 Bruce B. Downs Boulevard, Tampa, FL 33612, USA

Bales, K.R.
Neuroscience Discovery Research, Lilly Research Laboratories,
Indianapolis, IN 46285, USA

Bard, F.
Elan Pharmaceuticals
800 Gateway Blvd, South San Francisco, CA 94080, USA,
e-mail: fbard@elanpharma.com

Burton, D.R.
Department of Immunology and Molecular Biology,
The Scripps Research Institute, La Jolla, CA 92037, USA

Cao, C.
Dept. of Medical Microbiology and Immunology,
University of South Florida College of Medicine,
MDC 10, 12901 Bruce B. Downs Boulevard, Tampa, FL 33612, USA

Clements, J.D.
Department of Microbiology and Immunology,
Program in Molecular and Pathogenesis and Immunity,
Tulane University School of Medicine, New Orleans, LA 70112, USA

DeMattos, R.B.
Center for the Study of Nervous System Injury,
Alzheimer's Disease Research Center, Dept. of Neurology,

Washington University School of Medicine,
660 S. Euclid Ave., Box 811, St. Louis, MO 63110, USA

Dickey, C.
Alzheimer Research Laboratory, Department of Pharmacology,
University of South Florida College of Medicine,
12901 Bruce B. Downs Boulevard, Tampa, FL 33612, USA

Fraser, P.
Centre for Research in Neurodegenerative Disease, University of Toronto,
6 Queen's Park Crescent West, Toronto, Ontario M9B 5K3, Canada

Gordon, M.N.
Alzheimer Research Laboratory, Department of Pharmacology,
University of South Florida College of Medicine,
12901 Bruce B. Downs Boulevard, Tampa, FL 33612, USA

Holtzman, D.M.
Center for the Study of Nervous System Injury,
Alzheimer's Disease Research Center,
Dept. of Neurology, Molecular Biology and Pharmacology,
Washington University School of Medicine, 660 S. Euclid Ave., Box 811,
St. Louis, MO 63110, USA, e-mail: holtzman@neuro.wustl.edu

Hyman, B.T.
Massachusetts General Hospital/Harvard Medical School,
Department of Neurology, 115, 16th Street (CAGN 2009), Charlestown, MA 02129,
USA, e-mail: B_Hyman@helix.mgh.harvard.edu

Janus, C.
Centre for Research in Neurodegenerative Disease, University of Toronto,
6 Queen's Park Crescent West, Toronto, Ontario M9B 5K3, Canada

Johnson, H.-S.
Centre for Research in Neurodegenerative Disease, University of Toronto,
6 Queen's Park Crescent West, Toronto, Ontario M9B 5K3, Canada

Kaneko, K.
National Institute of Neuroscience, Tokyo 187-8502, Japan

Lemere, C.A.
Center for Neurologic Diseases, Brigham & Women's Hospital,
Harvard Medical School, Boston, MA 02115, USA,
e-mail: lemere@cnd.bwh.harvard.edu

Leverone, J.F.
Center for Neurologic Diseases, Brigham & Women's Hospital,
Harvard Medical School, Boston, MA 02115, USA

McLaurin, J.
Centre for Research in Neurodegenerative Disease, University of Toronto,
6 Queen's Park Crescent West, Toronto, Ontario M9B 5K3, Canada

Monsonego, A.
Center for Neurologic Diseases, Brighman and Women's Hospital,
Harvard Medical School, 77 Ave. Louis Pasteur, Boston, MA 02115, USA,
e-mail shoulder@rics.bwh.harvard.edu

Morgan, D.
Alzheimer Research Laboratory, Department of Pharmacology,
University of South Florida College of Medicine,
12901 Bruce B. Downs Boulevard, Tampa, FL 33612, USA

Paul, S.M.
Neuroscience Discovery Research, Lilly Research Laboratories,
Indianapolis, IN 46285, USA

Peretz, D.
Institute for Neurodegenerative Diseases and Departement of Neurology,
University of California, San Francisco, CA 94143-0518, USA,
e-mail: peretz@cgl.ucsf.edu

Prusiner, S.B.
Institute for Neurodegenerative Diseases and Departements of Neurology
and Biochemistry and Biophysics, University of California, San Francisco,
CA 94143-0518, USA

Schenk, D.
Elan Pharmaceuticals, 800 Gateway Blvd, South San Francisco, CA 94080, USA

Selkoe, D.J.
Center for Neurologic Diseases, Harvard Medical School and Brigham
and Women's Hospital, 77 Avenue Louis Pasteur, HIM 730, Boston, MA 02115,
USA, e-mail: dselkoe@rics.bwh.harvard.edu

Seubert, P.
Elan Pharmaceuticals, 800 Gateway Blvd, South San Francisco, CA 94080, USA

Solomon, B.
Department of Molecular Microbiology & Biotechnology,
George S. Wise Faculty of Life Sciences, Tel-Aviv University, Ramat Aviv,
Tel-Aviv, Israel 69978, e-mail: beka@post.tau.ac.il

Spooner, E.T.
Center for Neurologic Diseases, Brigham & Women's Hospital,
Harvard Medical School, Boston, MA 02115, USA

St.George-Hyslop, P.
Centre for Research in Neurodegenerative Disease, University of Toronto,
6 Queen's Park Crescent West, Toronto, Ontario M9B 5K3, Canada

Ugen, K.E.
Dept. of Medical Microbiology and Immunology,
University of South Florida College of Medicine, MDC 10,
12901 Bruce B. Downs Boulevard, Tampa, FL 33612, USA,
e-mail: kugen@hsc.usf.edu

Weiner, H.L.
Center for Neurologic Diseases, Brighman and Women's Hospital,
Harvard Medical School, 77 Ave. Louis Pasteur, Boston, MA 02115, USA,
e-mail: shoulder@rics.bwh.harvard.edu

Westaway, D.
Centre for Research in Neurodegenerative Disease, University of Toronto,
6 Queen's Park Crescent West, Toronto, Ontario M9B 5K3, Canada,
e-mail: .david.westaway@utoronto.ca

Wilcock, D.
Alzheimer Research Laboratory, Department of Pharmacology,
University of South Florida College of Medicine,
12901 Bruce B. Downs Boulevard, Tampa, FL 33612, USA

Williamson, R.A.,
Department of Immunology and Molecular Biology,
The Scripps Research Institute, La Jolla, CA 92037, USA

Yednock, T.
Elan Pharmaceuticals, 800 Gateway Blvd, South San Francisco, CA 94080, USA

Immunologic and Tolerogenic Aspects of Amyloid Beta-Peptide: Implications for the Pathogenesis and Treatment of Alzheimer's Disease

A. Monsonego[1] and H. L. Weiner[1]

Summary

Alzheimer's disease (AD) is marked by the progressive accumulation of amyloid beta-peptide (Aβ), which appears to trigger neurotoxic and inflammatory cascades. We investigated microglia as Aβ antigen-presenting cells (APCs) and their interaction with Aβ-reactive T-cells, as a potential cascade in AD pathology. We found that IFN-γ-treated microglia were potent Aβ APCs measured by T-cell reactivity to Aβ1-40 and Aβ1-42, the major accumulating peptides. In B6SJL mice transgenic for human APP under the prion promoter, chronic Aβ accumulation in the circulation was associated with immune hyporesponsiveness, apparently due to the lack of T-cell help for antibody production. In preliminary studies in humans, we have identified Aβ-reactive T-cells in peripheral blood lymphocytes with a stronger response seen to Aβ1-42 than to Aβ1-40. Taken together, our results suggest that Aβ-reactive T-cells exist in humans and, depending on genetic background, may expand in response to Aβ deposition in the brain and/or neurodegenerative cascades during aging. Further investigation of these endogenous immune responses to Aβ in humans may determine whether they contribute to, or protect against, AD and also whether they are involved in immunological reactions to Aβ vaccines used to treat AD.

Introduction

Brain injury such as occurs in trauma and in Alzheimer's Disease (AD) may evoke different classes of immune responses. There may be innate immune responses, characterized by astroglyosis and microgliosis, which can be associated with neurodegeneration (Tan et al. 1999; Bradt et al. 19998; Cooper et al. 2000). In addition, there are adaptive autoimmune responses in which brain-specific, T-cell and B-cell reactivity may be triggered. Adaptive immune responses are known to occur to self-antigens and are responsible for autoimmune diseases such as multiple sclerosis and diabetes (Ota et al. 1990; Wang et al. 1996). Nonetheless, adaptive immune responses can be beneficial to the host by generating regulatory cells and/or effector cells that may serve to clear pathogenic molecules or cells (Cohen and

[1] Center for Neurologic Diseases, Brigham and Women's Hospital, Harvard Medical School. 77 Ave. Louis Pasteur, Boston, MA 02115

Selkoe/Christen
Immunization Against Alzheimer's Disease
and Other Neurodegenerative Disorders
© Springer-Verlag Berlin Heidelberg 2003

Schwartz 1999; Schwartz and Cohen 2000; Zhang et al. 2001). Naive T-cells can differentiate into different sub-classes depending on cytokine milieu and the antigen itself. TH1 type cells are generated in the context of IL-12 and function to clear bacteria and viruses and may be pathogenic if reacted to self-antigens. TH-2 and TH-3 T-cells are favorably generated at mucosal surfaces and involve differentiation factors such as IL-4 and IL-10. These cells secrete IL-4, IL-10, and TGF-β, which can down regulate autoimmune responses and may be beneficial to the host.

AD is associated with increased production and deposition of amyloid beta-peptide (Aβ) in the brain (Selkoe 1998). A chronic, innate immune response is associated with Aβ plaques and appears to induce further neuronal loss (Cooper et al. 2000; McGeer and McGeer 1998). Under these circumstances Aβ can also serve as a self-antigen and be a target of an antigen's specific immune response. This cascade would have to involve interaction between CNS antigen-presenting cells (APCs) and peripheral Aβ-reactive T-cells. In our studies we characterized these two cellular components with regard to Aβ-mediated adaptive and humoral immune responses.

Microglia as Aβ-Antigen Presenting Cells

To generate an adaptive immune response, an antigen must be phagocytosed and processed by professional APCs. In the central nervous system microglia serve as the major APCs that can express significant amounts of MHC class II and the costimulatory molecules needed to evoke T-cell activation (Aloisi 2001). We generated primary cultures of glial cells from one-day-old mice and stimulated them with IFN-γ for 72 hours. CD11b+/CD11c+ microglia were sorted (Fig. 1A) and cocultured with Aβ-reactive T-cells for 48 hours. We found that IFN-γ-treated microglia served as excellent Aβ APCs, as indicated by Aβ-reactive T-cell proliferation (Fig. 1B). Astrocytes were also shown to have APC characteristics when treated with different stimulators such as IFN-γ. To test their ability to stimulate Aβ-reactive T-cells, we first enriched the astrocytes population by shaking the glial cultures for 24 hours and then sorted all CD11b+ cells. This procedure removes most of the microglia and oligodendrocytes from the culture. Astrocytes were then cultured alone or in the presence of microglia and were incubated with IFN-γ for 72 hours, followed by co-culturing with Aβ-reactive T-cells. Astrocytes alone could not induce Aβ-reactive T-cell proliferation (Fig. 1B). Moreover, microglia-mediated T-cell proliferation was substantially reduced when cocultured with astrocytes (Fig. 1B). Since Aβ1-42 tends to fibrillate very rapidly and, therefore, may be less vulnerable for processing by microglia, we tested whether Aβ fibrillation affected Aβ-reactive T-cell proliferation. As shown in Figure 1C, T-cell proliferation was more abundant with the fibrillated forms of both Aβ1-40 and Aβ1-42 compared with the soluble forms.

In summary, Aβ deposition may trigger microglial activation, which results in the secretion of TNF-α, IL-1β, IL-6, complement, and NO, all of which are factors that may lead to neurotoxicity. In the presence of IFN-γ, microglia can differentiate into APCs and stimulate effector and/or regulatory Aβ-reactive T-cells that may lead to more efficient clearance of Aβ and, ultimately, potential neuroprotection.

Fig. 1. IFN-γ-treated microglia induce proliferation of Aβ-reactive T-cells. Glial cultures were prepared as follows: cells were dissociated from the cerebral cortex of 1-day-old C57BL/6 mice, while carefully removing meninges tissue, and were cultured in poly-D-lysine (PDL)-coated tissue culture flasks. At day 10 CD11b⁺/CD11c⁺ microglial and glial cells (CD11b-) were sorted (**a**), and then cocultured with resting Aβ-reactive T-cells (5×10^4/well) in the presence and absence of Aβ1-42. Aβ-reactive T-cell proliferation was measured at 72 hours after stimulation with microglia alone, glial cells alone, or in combination (**b**). Aβ1-40 or Aβ1-42 were fibrillated for three days at 37° C and were used as antigens to measure T-cell proliferation (**c**).

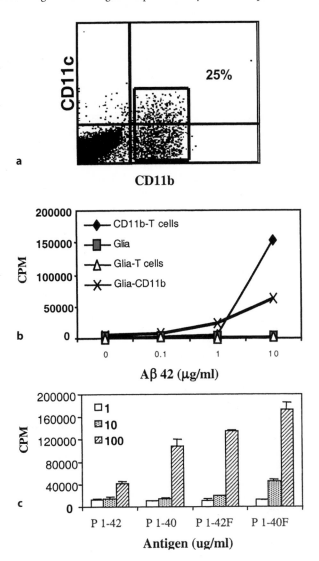

Aβ-Mediated immune Hyporesponsiveness in APP-Tg Mice

A growing body of evidence has demonstrated that self-reactive lymphocytes may escape negative selection or may even be positively selected to be part of the normal immune repertoire (Janeway 1999). Since Aβ associates with pathology in the CNS, it may involve the activation and expansion of Aβ-reactive T-cells. Nonetheless, antigen itself is a primary driving factor in immune tolerance, and it has been shown that exposure of soluble antigen in the thymus induces tolerance (Peterson et al. 1999). Immunologic tolerance involves multiple mechanisms by which self-reactive lymphocytes cannot cause harm to the host. In APP-Tg mice there is high expression of human APP in the brain and substantial levels of human Aβ in the serum. Thus, this finding raises the question of whether the chronic expression of Aβ in the brain and the levels of APP in the blood may lead to hyporesponsiveness of Aβ-reactive T- or B-cells. This is an important question, given that there is an interest in treating AD by generating adaptive immune responses to Aβ. To address the question of adaptive immune responses in these animals, APP-Tg mice were immunized with Aβ peptide and then immune responses were studied. We found that Aβ antibody production was suppressed in APP-Tg mice compared with non-transgenic littermates (Fig. 2). We also observed a decrease in Aβ-induced T-cell proliferation and cytokine production (Fig. 3). To investigate whether this tolerance was related to T-cell or B-cell tolerance, we conjugated the B-cell epitope Aβ1-15 to BSA as a carrier and immunized APP-Tg mice. We found that immunization with BSA-conjugated Aβ1-15 induced

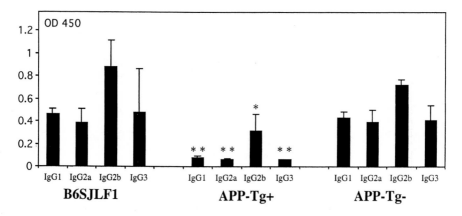

Fig. 2. Suppressed anti-Aβ antibody production in immunized APP-Tg+mice. Control B6SJL, APP-Tg+ and APP-Tg- mice were immunized with Aβ1-40 at five weeks of age and analyzed 10 days later for anti-Aβ antibody production. IgG1, IgG2a, IgG2b and IgG3 anti-Aβ antibodies were measured by ELISA for APP-tg+ (n=7) and APP-Tg- (n=7) littermates as well as for control wild-type mice (n=6). The data shown are for sera dilution of 1:100, as a higher dilution did not yield detection of significant anti-Aβ antibodies in the APP-Tg+ animals. All isotypes are significantly decreased in the APP-Tg+ mice compared with APP-Tg- (*p<0.0001, ** p<0.0005).

Fig. 3. Decreased Aβ-induced T-cell proliferation and cytokine production. APP-Tg+ and APP-Tg- mice were immunized with Aβ1-40. In vitro T-cell proliferation induced by either Aβ1-40 or Aβ1-42 was measured after incubating by the lymph node-derived lymphocytes with the respective Aβ peptide for three days, followed by 3H-thymidine incorporation for 12 h. Stimulation index (S.I.) represents the CPM in the presence of antigen divided by the CPM in the absence of antigen. T-cells from the various groups were also tested for Aβ-mediated cytokine secretion. Results are shown for Aβ-induced IL-2 and IFN-γ production measured at 24 and 40 h after Aβ stimulation, respectively.

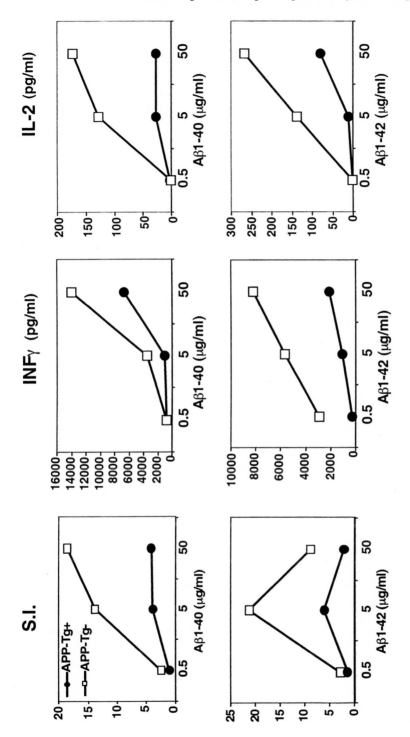

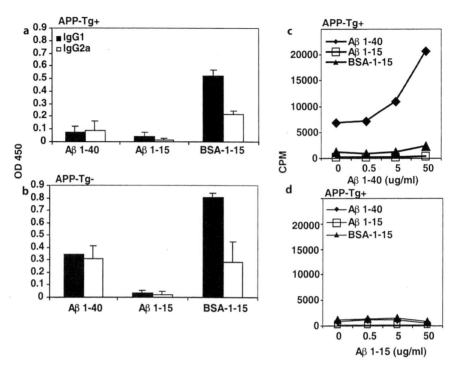

Fig. 4. Immunization with BSA-conjugated Aβ 1-15 induces high titers of anti-Aβ antibodies in APP-Tg+ mice. APP-Tg littermates (both + and –) were immunized with one of the following antigens: Aβ1-40, Aβ1-15, or BSA-conjugated Aβ1-15. At day 10 post-immunization, mice were bled and PLN were excised. Titers of IgG1 and IgG2a anti-Aβ1-40 antibodies were measured in the serum of the APP-Tg+ (**a**) and APP-Tg– (**b**) littermates by ELISA. In addition PLN-derived cells from APP-Tg+ mice were stimulated in vitro at day 10 post-immunization with either Aβ1-4o (**c**) or Aβ1-15 (**d**) for a T-cell proliferation assay. Note that levels of Aβ were measured by ELISA in pre-immune sera of the APP-Tg+ mice tested, and the concentrations were found to be similar for the Aβ1-40 group (576.6±117 pg/ml), the Aβ1-15 group (540±198 pg/ml), and the BSA-conjugated Aβ1-15 group (616.6±231 pg/ml).

high titers of antibodies to Aβ in these mice (Fig. 4). The immune hyporesponsiveness could be overcome if T-cell help was provided by coupling an Aβ B-cell epitope to BSA. These results suggest that overexpression of APP in mice is associated with an Aβ-specific, impaired adaptive immune response that may contribute to the neuropathology. Furthermore, humans with life-long elevation of Aβ in the brain and the periphery could have reduced immune responses to Aβ vaccination. Our results demonstrate that chronic pre-symptomatic accumulation of Aβ in the brain may make it more difficult to induce antibody responses in such patients and that coupling the B-cell epitope to a carrier could obviate this problem. Such an immunization paradigm would preferentially induce antibody responses and minimal Aβ-reactive T-cell responses.

Immune Responses to Aβ in Humans

Any immune-based therapy in AD must take into account T-cell reactivity to Aβ. T-cell reactivity may have been responsible for the encephalitis that was observed in patients immunized with Aβ 1-42 in a recent trial conducted by Elan Pharmaceutical. Furthermore, differential T-cell reactivity may have implications for the development of AD in individual patients and the degree to which the disease progresses. To investigate T-cell responses in Alzheimer's patients, we carried out a split-well assay in which the peripheral blood mononuclear cells (PBMCs) were isolated from young and old individuals and cultured with Aβ. Cells were cultured for ten days, after which each well was split and re-cultured in the presence and absence of Aβ. Using this technique, we identified Aβ reactivity as measured by T-cell proliferation in the presence and absence of Aβ. Aβ-reactive T-cells were measured in young individuals (age 30-40) using Aβ1-42 as antigen. Sixteen percent of the wells showed a stimulation index of 3 or higher and a Δcpm higher than 10,000 in a representative blood sample (Fig. 5). In a preliminary experiment, results suggested greater reactivity in older individuals. These results suggest that reactivity to Aβ may increase with age and could contribute to the disease process. We are in the process of characterizing human Aβ reactive T-cell lines in terms of epitope specificity, responsiveness, and cytokine pattern.

Differential T-cell reactivity could be very important and could explain the encephalitis that was observed with immunization of Alzheimer's patients. In the model of EAE induced with MOG peptides we observed that SJL mice were susceptible to EAE whereas B 10.S mice were resistant (Maron et al. 1999). The susceptibility and resistance of these animals were related to the class of T-cell response that was generated. The SJL animals had increased amounts of IFN-γ relative to B10.S and minimal secretion of IL-10 or TGF-β. On the other hand B10.S animals secreted less IFN-γ and more IL-10 and TGF-β. These findings were associated with expression of IL-4 and TGF-β in the brains of B10.S mice and not in the brains of SJL mice. This differential class of immune response was also observed in our study of nasal immunization of APP-Tg mice. Namely, Th2 type of antibodies and infiltration of small numbers of IL-4, IL-10 and TGF-β-secreting cells were observed in the APP-Tg mice (Weiner et al. 2000). Thus one might postulate that the mucosal administration of Aβ may induce antibodies but preferentially induce T-cells, which are non-pathogenic. Factors that may influence a class of immune response include route of antigen exposure, type of antigen, the genetics of the host, and the adjuvant used. All of these factors may be crucial in developing an Aβ vaccination that is not harmful to the host.

Aβ 1-42 (40 ug/ml)

-	+	-	+	-	+	-	+	-	+
43789	37865	45099	48685	35245	21634	8745	69821	45723	142880
173254	141713	11392	85226	16037	22330	36315	38569	63579	50010
19889	20689	64853	33523	13687	11926	12871	56147	50468	46617
5874	5566	26719	57697	41186	31531	25355	19537	18268	16304
18923	30122	23614	35242	15753	19795	78577	35267	164315	150771
18816	17705	15029	24260	7300	8183	67300	78350	1542	427

Fig. 5. In vitro stimulation of blood-derived Aβ-reactive T-cells. PBMCs were purified from blood using Percol gradient centrifugation and were cultured in 30 wells of U-bottom 96 well plates in the presence of Aβ. On day 10, cells were analyzed by means of the split-well assay: half the cells from each well were restimulated with irradiated PBMCs in the presence and absence of Aβ for 48 hours and were then pulsed with [³H] thymidine for 12 hours. Cells were then harvested and radioactivity was measured (cpm). The stimulation index (cpm in the presence of Aβ divided by cpm in the absence of Aβ) was determined. Positive wells were those with a stimulation index of ≥ 3 and a delta cpm ≥ 10,000.

Conclusion

As shown in Figure 6, Aβ accumulation can lead directly to neurotoxicity. Furthermore it may activate microglia that, through the innate immune response and the secretion TNF-α and IL-1β, can augment the neurotoxicty. The activation of microglia by IFN-γ may also lead to the presentation of Aβ by microglia in the context of MHC, which can then stimulate adaptive immune responses. These adaptive immune responses may be enhanced or deficient depending on mechanisms of tolerance (Monsonego et al. 2001) and the genetic background of the individual. Furthermore, these adaptive immune responses may be beneficial in decreasing Aβ accumulation and microglial activation. On the other hand, adaptive immune responses may be detrimental, as was presumably observed in the encephalitis that occurred following Aβ immunization with an adjuvant in humans, which presumably led to activation of pathogenic, disease-inducing T-cells.

It is clear that a detailed understanding of immune responses to Aβ, both innate and adaptive, will be required to successfully apply immunization strategies for the treatment of the disease. Nonetheless, given what has been observed to date, it appears that these strategies can ultimately be effective in patients, given that the appropriate immune responses are generated and the immune repertoire of the individuals being vaccinated is well defined.

In our center we are considering a trial of mucosal administered Aβ and the possibility of utilizing adjuvants that will drive TH2 as opposed to TH1 responses. In addition, we are in the process of characterizing immune responses to Aβ in young and old individuals and attempting to link such responses to the expression of AD and its severity.

Fig. 6. From Aβ to neurotoxicity. Aβ accumulation can lead directly to neurotoxicity. It may also activate microglia that can augment toxicity and stimulate adaptive immune responses which may be beneficial.

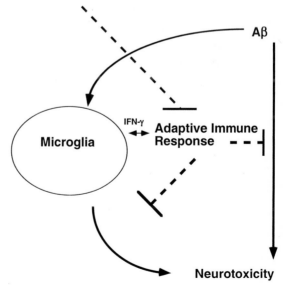

References

1 Aloisi F (2001) Immune function of microglia. Glia 36:165–179
2 Bradt BM, Kolb WP, Cooper NR (1998) Complement-dependent proinflammatory properties of the Alzheimer's disease beta-peptide. J Exp Med 188:431–438
3 Cohen IR, Schwartz M (1999) Autoimmune maintenance and neuroprotection of the central nervous system. J Neuroimmunol 100:111–114
4 Cooper NR, Kalaria RN, McGeer PL, Rogers J (2000) Key issues in Alzheimer's disease inflammation. Neurobiol Aging 21:451–453
5 Janeway CA Jr (1999) T-cell development: a role for self-peptides in positive selection. Curr Biol 9:R 342–345
6 Maron R, Hancock WW, Slavin A, Hattori M, Kuchroo V, Weiner HL (1999) Genetic susceptibility or resistance to autoimmune encephalomyelitis in MHC congenic mice is associated with differential production of pro- and anti-inflammatory cytokines. Int Immunol 11:1573–1580
7 McGeer EG, McGeer PL (1998) The importance of inflammatory mechanisms in Alzheimer disease. Exp Gerontol 33:371–378
8 Monsonego A, Maron R, Zota V, Selkoe DJ, Weiner HL (2001) Immune hyporesponsiveness to amyloid beta-peptide in amyloid precursor protein transgenic mice: implications for the pathogenesis and treatment of Alzheimer's disease. Proc Natl Acad Sci USA 98:10273–10278
9 Ota K, Matsui M, Milford EL, Mackin GA, Weiner HL, Hafler DA (1990) T-cell recognition of an immunodominant myelin basic protein epitope in multiple sclerosis. Nature 346:183–187
10 Peterson DA, DiPaolo RJ, Kanagawa O, Unanue ER (1999) Quantitative analysis of the T-cell repertoire that escapes negative selection. Immunity 11:453–463
11 Schwartz M, Cohen IR (2000) Autoimmunity can benefit self-maintenance [In Process Citation]. Immunol Today 21:265–268
12 Selkoe DJ (1998) The cell biology of beta-amyloid precursor protein and presenilin in Alzheimer's disease. Trends Cell Biol 8:447–453
13 Tan J, Town T, Paris D, Mori T, Suo Z, Crawford F, Mattson MP, Flavell RA, Mullan M (1999) Microglial activation resulting from CD40-CD40L interaction after beta-amyloid stimulation. Science 286:2352–2355
14 Wang B, Gonzalez A, Benoist C, Mathis D (1996) The role of CD8+ T-cells in the initiation of insulin-dependent diabetes mellitus. Eur J Immunol 26:1762–1769
15 Weiner HL, Lemere CA, Maron R, Spooner ET, Grenfell TJ, Mori C, Issazadeh S, Hancock WW, Selkoe DJ (2000) Nasal administration of amyloid-beta peptide decreases cerebral amyloid burden in a mouse model of Alzheimer's disease. Ann Neurol 48:567–579
16 Zhang X, Izikson L, Liu L, Weiner HL (2001) Activation of CD25(+)CD4(+) regulatory T-cells by oral antigen administration. J Immunol 167:4245–4253

Towards Diagnosis and Treatment of Alzheimer's Disease

B. Solomon[1]

Summary

More and more evidence shows that Alzheimer's disease belongs to the family of conformational diseases characterized by protein self-association and tissue deposition as amyloid fibrils. As recently shown, monoclonal antibodies interact at strategic sites where conformational changes of proteins are initiated, stabilizing the protein and preventing further aggregation. These data, and the recent performance of such antibodies in transgenic mice as a model for human diseases, convert the immunological concept into a therapeutic strategy for the development of vaccination against such diseases. Here we describe a new immunization procedure against β-amyloid plaques using as antigen the EFRH peptide displayed on the surface of the filamentous phage. Antibodies to the epitope EFRH, representing residues 3–6 within the β-amyloid peptide, were found to modulate its in vitro solubility and aggregation. The EFRH phage induced effective anti-aggregating antibodies in transgenic mice that recapitulate the amyloid plaques and vascular pathology of Alzheimer's disease. The immunization led to a considerable reduction in the number of β-amyloid plaques found in the brains of the sacrificed transgenic mice. However, effective means are required for in vivo brain imaging to monitor changes in the plaque burden of patients' brains. We propose anti-β-amyloid antibodies displayed on genetically engineered filamentous phages as a specific probe to monitor amyloid plaque formation in living patients. Intranasal administration of filamentous phage as a delivery vector of anti-β-amyloid antibody fragment into brains of Alzheimer's APP transgenic mice enables in vivo targeting of β-amyloid plaques. The plaques were co-visualized both by Thioflavin-S and fluorescent-labeled antibodies in the olfactory bulb and hippocampal regions, which correlate with early plaque formation. The genetically engineered filamentous bacteriophage proved to be an efficient and non-toxic viral delivery vector to the brain, offering an obvious advantage over mammalian vectors. Future studies will determine if coupling-up radiopharmaceuticals to phage carrying antibodies would detect brain amyloid deposits in vivo. The feasibility of these novel strategies may have clinical potential for diagnosis and treatment of Alzheimer's disease and other brain disorders.

---

[1] Department of Molecular Microbiology & Biotechnology, George S. Wise Faculty of Life Sciences, Tel-Aviv University, Ramat Aviv, Tel-Aviv, Israel 69978

Selkoe/Christen
Immunization Against Alzheimer's Disease
and Other Neurodegenerative Disorders
© Springer-Verlag Berlin Heidelberg 2003

Introduction

The association of protein deposits with neurodegeneration has become a consistent finding in a large group of etiologically diverse diseases. The protein deposits – β amyloids – are generally dense fibrillar structures containing a high percentage of β-pleat sheet secondary structure and can be located variously in cellular and extracellular compartments (Wetzel 1994; Kaytor and Warren 1999). Despite the diverse nature of the precursor proteins involved in amyloid formation, all amyloid fibrils have characteristic physicochemical, tinctorial and ultrastructural features. Understanding the mechanisms and molecular details of conformational conversion may help in developing approaches for prevention and treatment of such cases.

Recently, the immunological concept in the treatment of conformational diseases has been converted into a therapeutic strategy for Alzheimer's disease (AD) treatment (Solomon 2001). Antibody-antigen interactions involve conformational changes in both antibody and antigen that can range from insignificant to considerable. Binding of high affinity monoclonal antibodies (mAbs) to regions of high flexibility and antigenicity may alter the molecular dynamics of the whole antigen (Frauenfelder et al. 1979; Karplus and Petsko 1990). Experimental data show that mAbs are able to stabilize the antigen by preventing aggregation and resolubilizing already formed protein aggregates (Solomon and Ballas, 1991; Katzav-Golansky et al. 1996). Moreover, monoclonal antibodies were found to recognize an incompletely folded epitope and induce native conformation in a partially unfolded protein (Blond and Goldberg 1987; Carlson and Yarmush 1992; Solomon and Schwartz 1995). For such an active role, the mAbs require a high binding constant to the "strategic" positions on the antigen molecule. In addition, such antibodies should be non-inhibitory to the biological activity of the respective antigen.

Immunomodulation of Amyloid Formation

The conformational state of β-amyloid peptide (AβP) has been reported to be a crucial factor in its neurotoxic activity in vitro, and possibly in vivo (Iversen et al. 1995; Small et al. 2001). How AβP form fibrils in vivo is not yet completely clear, but the process of fibril formation has been extensively studied in vitro (Clippingdale et al. 2001). Amyloid filaments, similar to those found in amyloid plaques and cerebrovascular amyloid, can be assembled from chemically synthesized β-peptide under well-defined experimental conditions in vitro, and the effect on neural cells may be neurotoxic or neurotrophic, depending on the β-amyloid (Aβ) fibrillar state (Lorenzo and Yankner 1994; Howlett et al. 1995). In vitro amyloid formation is a complex kinetic and thermodynamic process and the reversibility of amyloid plaque growth in vitro suggests a steady-state equilibrium between AβP in plaques and in solution (Maggio and Mantyh 1996). AβP can adopt two alternative conformations depending on the secondary structure of the amino-terminal domain (Soto 1999). The carboxy-terminal invariably adopts a β-sheet secondary structure in aqueous solution, whereas the amino-terminal domain shows either a β-sheet or α-helical secondary structure depending on environmental conditions (Kirshenbaum and Daggett 1995; Lee et al. 1995). It has been demonstrated that the secondary structure adopted by the amino-terminal can determine the propensity of AβP to aggregate (Lee et al. 1995). It has also been reported that amino-terminal deletions enhance aggregation of AβP in vitro (Pike et al. 1995). Artificial mutants that favor the α-helical structure considerably decrease the aggregation ability of the peptide; however, mutations favoring the β-sheet conformation have a higher propensity to aggregate, as seen with the Dutch mutation of APP (Soto et al. 1995).

The transition of the α-helix to β-sheet conformation with concomitant peptide aggregation is the proposed mechanism of plaque formation. The dependence of AβP polymerization on peptide-peptide interactions to form a β-pleated sheet fibril and the stimulatory influence of other proteins on the reaction suggest that amyloid formation may be subject to modulation. The perturbations in the equilibrium of various conformational states of AβP, leading to its amyloid pathological state, can be caused by various factors, genetic and environmental, as local pH changes, or by other proteins that act as pathological "chaperones" and accelerate the formation of Aβ fibril by binding to the N-terminal of the AβP (Talafous et al.1994). If so-called pathological chaperones like ApoE and heparan sulfate, increase the extent of β-amyloid formation (Wisniewski et al. 1994), we propose site-directed monoclonal antibodies against β-amyloid peptides, which decrease β-amyloid formation, as therapeutic chaperones.

We investigated a large panel of mAbs against various regions of AβP and found that only mAbs targeting the N-terminal regions, namely 6C6 and 10D5, of the β-peptide exhibit anti-aggregating properties. Binding of such antibodies interfered with noncovalent interactions between the amyloid fibrils and led to deterioration of amyloid fibrillar assembly into an amorphous form, even at antibody-peptide molar ratios of 1:100. The prevention of peptide aggregation, as well as the solubilization of already formed aggregates, required an equimolar ratio of Aβ-peptide, indicating the molecular level of these interactions (Solomon et al. 1996, 1997; Hanan and Solomon 1996).

Using phage-peptide libraries, composed of filamentous phage displaying random combinatorial peptides, we defined the EFRH residues located at positions 3-6 of the N-terminal AβP as the epitope of anti-aggregating antibodies 6C6 and 10D5 within AβP (Frenkel et al. 1998). The EFRH epitope is available for antibody binding when the β-amyloid peptide is either in solution or is an aggregate, and locking of this epitope by antibodies affects the dynamics of all the molecules, preventing self-aggregation as well as enabling resolubilization of already formed aggregates. Identification of the epitope of another antibody, namely mAb 2H3, which binds to the N-terminal of β-amyloid, highlights the importance of this specific sequence region, defined as an anti-aggregating epitope, on the behavior of the whole AβP molecule (Frenkel et al. 1999). Further research showed that the EFRH peptide strongly inhibits binding of anti-aggregating mAbs 6C6 and 10D5 to AβP (10^7M) but weakly inhibits binding of mAb 2H3 to AβP (10^{-4}M). Mab 2H3, which recognizes EFRH with a lower binding constant, showed an insignificant effect on the disruption of the β-amyloid fibrils already formed (Solomon et al. 1997).

It can be assumed that the epitope EFRH, located at the soluble tail of the N-terminal region, is involved in the aggregation process and acts as a regulatory site controlling both the solubilization and the disaggregation process of the AβP molecule. Locking of the EFRH epitope by highly specific antibodies affects the dynamics of the entire AβP molecule, preventing self-aggregation as well as res-olubilization of already formed aggregates. Moreover, the interaction of this epi-tope with such specific antibodies may interfere with pathological mechanisms in AD.

Clearance of β-Amyloid Plaques by EFRH-Phage Immunization

The abundant evidence that AβP aggregation is an essential early event in AD pathogenesis has prompted an intensive search for therapeutics that target Aβ. This search has been aided immeasurably by transgenic mouse models of AD. Several labs have bred AD diseased models of transgenic mice that produce Aβ and develop plaques and neuron damage in their brains (as reviewed inVan Leu-ven 2000). Although they do not develop the widespread neuron death and severe dementia seen in the human disease, they are used as models for the study of AD.

The immunization approach has a great impact on fibril formation in trans-genic mice and thus becomes a legitimate therapeutic approach. However, it seems to face many obstacles before being efficient in humans.

Several therapeutic strategies in vaccination against β-amyloid have recently been reported (Schenk et al. 1999; Bard et al. 2000; Sigurdsson et al. 2001; Lemere et al. 2001; DeMattos et al. 2001). We developed an immunization procedure for raising anti-AβP antibodies using as antigen the only EFRH peptide displayed on the filamentous phage. We have shown that immunization with a filamentous bacteriophage, carrying about 300 copies of the EFRH epitope, elicited high titers of IgG antibodies with high affinity against the Aβ peptide in a relatively short period of time (Frenkel et al. 2000a). The anti-EFRH-phage antisera were demon-strated to label the amyloid plaques effectively, both in brain sections of human AD patients and in brain sections of the transgenic mice. These antibodies were operationally similar or identical in their in vitro and in vivo anti-aggregating properties to antibodies raised by injection of whole AβP (Frenkel et al. 2000a, 2001; Solomon and Frenkel, 2000).

Clearance of β-amyloid plaques in vivo was demonstrated using APP[717I] transgenic mice, aged 16 months (Moechars et al. 1996), immunized with the EFRH-phage and analyzed at age 21 months. At this age the amyloid plaque pathology is maximally and stably established. Age-matched APP[V717I] trans-genic mice were injected with vehicle only and served as untreated controls. All mice received four ip injections every two weeks followed by two booster injec-tions one and two months later – a total of six injections over four and a half months. Five of eight (65%) APP[V717I] transgenic mice that were immunized with the EFRH-phage developed and maintained serum titers of antibodies against Aβ that varied between 1:100-1:1000. Three (35%) of the APP[V717I] transgenic mice developed only a low titer (~1:10) over the five-month immu-nization period. The amyloid burden in the brain was significantly reduced in the immunized APP[V717I] transgenic mice that developed anti-Aβ titers of at least 1:100, indicating a dose-response relation between antibody titer and reduced amyloid load (Frenkel et al. submitted for publication).

The clinical trials of novel techniques to decrease the burden of amyloid plaques require reliable and sensitive methods to monitor plaque presence/disappearance in the brains of living AD patients. Accurate targeting of Aβ plaques in brain regions could allow the preventative treatment and monitoring of drug efficacy during and after those trials.

We propose filamentous bacteriophages as antibody brain delivery vectors. The filamentous phages M13, fl and fd, are well understood at both the structural

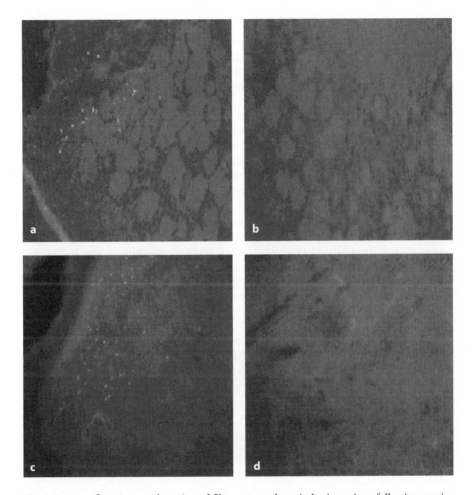

Fig. 1. Immunofluorescence detection of filamentous phage in brain regions following one intranasal administration. The presence of filamentous phage in mice olfactory bulb (**A**) and hippocampus sections (**C**) after one day and its disappearance after 28 days (**B, D**, respectively). The sections were observed on a fluorescence microscope at a final magnification of x 10.

and genetic levels (Greenwood et al. 1991) and offer an obvious advantage over mammalian vectors.

Intranasally administered filamentous phages were detected in both the olfactory bulb and hippocampal region (Frenkel et al. 2000b). We supposed that, due to its linear structure, the filamentous phage is highly permeable to different kinds of membranes and following the olfactory tracts it may reach the hippocampus regions (Fig. 1). Phages were not detected in the brain 28 days after administration, and several hypotheses may be considered regarding the disappearance of the filamentous phage from the brain without inducing any toxic effect. No visible toxic effects due to phage administration were detected in the treated animals. Histology studies showed no such effects, even after more than six months following treatment. (Frenkel and Solomon 2002).

The ability of filamentous phages to display and stabilize therapeutic molecules, such as small engineered antibodies (scFv), on their surface, together with their efficient entry into the CNS, was examined using an anti-β-amyloid antibody fragment scFv-508 fused to a filamentous minor coat peptide pIII.

The anti-β-amyloid scFv-phage targets in vivo β-amyloid plaques in APP transgenic mice (Frenkel and Solomon 2002). The β-amyloid plaques were co-visualized both by ThS and fluorescent-labeled anti-phage antibodies (Fig. 2). Following intranasal phage administration of scFv in these mice, β-amyloid brain plaques were specifically labeled in the two specific brain sections (olfactory and hippocampus) where most of the early amyloid plaques are located. (Naslund et al. 2000). The stained plaques show high sensitivity, similar to those from human AD patients detected in vitro by immunofluorescent techniques (Fig. 3).

The results confirmed the high specificity of scFv-phage for in vivo targeting of β-amyloid plaques. Future experiments will be performed to radiolabel anti-β-amyloid antibodies with an isotope more suitable for diagnostic imaging, like ^{123}I, and to test their ability to label and detect amyloid deposits in live transgenic mice.

Coupling of radiopharmaceuticals to phage antibodies and using one of the diagnostic imaging methods used in humans, such as single photon emission

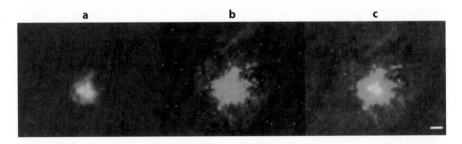

Fig. 2. a typical stained β-amyloid plaque from several others scanned with the fluorescent confocal microscope in vivo targeted by scFv display on filamentous phage. Beta-amyloid plaques in mouse hippocampus sections were detected both with Thioflavin-S staining in yellow (**a**) and anti-phage antibodies, represented in red (**b**); (**c**) represents double labeling of the plaques (scale bar: 5μm).

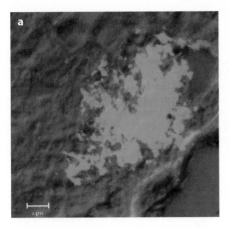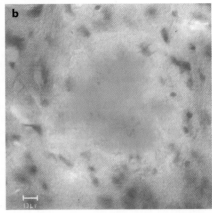

Fig. 3. Immunofluorescence detection of β-amyloid plaques by scFv in human AD affected brain sections. β-amyloid plaques in hippocampus sections of human Alzheimer's patients (**A**) detected by scFv displayed on filamentous phage were compared to Congo red staining (**B**). The sections were observed on a confocal microscope at a final magnification of x 66.

computed tomography (SPECT), may detect brain amyloid deposits, leading to an early and efficient diagnostic test for AD.

Conclusions

Monoclonal antibodies interact at strategic sites where conformational changes of proteins are initiated, stabilizing the protein and preventing further aggregation. These data, and the recent performance of such antibodies in transgenic mice as a model for human diseases, convert the immunological concept into a therapeutic strategy for vaccination against such diseases.

Indeed, the immunization approach seems to have great impact on the modulation of amyloid fibril formation in the transgenic mice model of human so-called "conformational" diseases.

In spite of the many obstacles that will have to be overcome before the efficient use of the immunological approach in disease-affected human patients, several active and passive approaches in the vaccination against Alzheimer's β-amyloid are being developed. Additional studies are needed and are ongoing towards early diagnosis of the disease and towards therapeutic intervention before cognitive decline occurs.

References

Bard F, Cannon C, Barbour R, Burke R-L, Games D, Grajeda H, Guido T, Hu K, Huang J, Johnson-Wood K, Khan K, Kholodenko D, Lee M, Lieberburg I, Motter R, Nguyen M, Soriano F, Vasquez N, Weiss K, Welch B, Seubert P, Schenk D, Yednock T (2000) Peripherally administered antibodies against amyloid beta-peptide enter the central nervous system and reduce pathology in a mouse model of Alzheimer disease. Nature Med 6: 916–920

Blond S, Goldberg M (1987) Partly native epitopes are already present on early intermediates in the folding of tryptophan synthase. Proc Natl Acad Sci USA 84: 1147–1151

Carlson JD, Yarmush ML (1992) Antibody assisted protein refolding. Biotechnology 10:86–91

Clippingdale AB, Wade JD, Barrow CY (2001) The amyloid-beta peptide and its role in Alzheimer's disease. J Pept Sci 7:227–249

DeMattos RB, Bales KR, Cummins DJ, Dodart JC, Paul SM, Holtzman DM (2001) Peripheral anti-Aβ antibody alters CNS and plasma Aβ clearance and decreases brain Aβ burden in a mouse model of Alzheimer's disease. Proc Natl Acad Sci USA 17: 8850-8855

Frauenfelder H, Petsko GA, Tsernoglou, D (1979) Temperature dependent x-ray diffraction as a probe of protein structural dynamics. Nature 280:558–563

Frenkel D, Solomon B (2002) Filamentous phage as vector-mediated antibody delivery to the brain. Proc Natl Acad Sci USA, 99:5675–5679

Frenkel D, Balass M, Solomon B (1998) N-terminal EFRH sequence of Alzheimer's β-amyloid peptide represents the epitope of its anti-aggregating antibodies. J Neuroimmunol 88:85–90

Frenkel D, Balass M, Kachalsky-Katzir E,.Solomon B (1999) High affinity binding of monoclonal antibodies to the sequential epitope EFRH of β-amyloid peptide is essential for modulation of fibrillar aggregation. J Neuroimmunol 95:136–142

Frenkel D, Katz O, Solomon B (2000a). Immunization against Alzheimer's β-amyloid plaques via EFRH phage administration. Proc Natl Acad Sci USA 97:11455–11459

Frenkel D, Solomon B, Benhar I (2000b) Modulation of Alzheimer's β-amyloid neurotoxicity by site-directed single-chain antibody. J Neuroimmunol 106:23–31

Frenkel D, Kariv N, Solomon B (2001) Generation of auto-antibodies towards Alzheimer's disease vaccination. Vaccine 19:2615–2619

Greenwood J, Willis EA, Perham NR (1991) Multiple display of foreign peptides on a filamentous bacteriophage. J Mol Biol 220: 821–827

Hanan E, Solomon B (1996) Inhibitory effect of monoclonal antibodies on Alzheimer's β-amyloid peptide aggregation. Amyloid: Int J Exp Clin Invest 3:130–133

Howlett DR, Jennings KH, Lee DC, Clark MSG, Brown F, Wetzel R, Wood SJ, Camilleri P, Roberts GW (1995) Aggregation state and neurotoxic properties of Alzheimer beta-amyloid peptide. Neurodegeneration 4: 23–32

Iversen LL, Mortishire-Smith RJ, Pollack SJ, Shearman MS (1995) The toxicity *in vitro* of beta-amyloid protein. Biochem J 311:1–16

Karplus M, Petsko GA (1990) Molecular dynamics simulations in biology. Nature 347: 631–639

Katzav-Gozansky T, Hanan E, Solomon B (1996) Effect of monoclonal antibodies in preventing carboxypeptidase A aggregation. Biotechnol Appl Biochem 23:227–230

Kaytor MD, Warren ST (1999) Aberrant protein deposition and neurological disease. J Biol Chem 31:37507–35710

Kirshenbaum K, Daggett V (1995) PH-dependent conformations of the amyloid beta (1-28) peptide fragment explored using molecular dynamics. Biochemistry 34:7629–7639

Lee JP, Stimson ER, Ghilardi JR, Mantyh PW, Lu YA, Felix AM, Llanos W, Behbin A, Cummings M, Van Criekinge M, Timms W, Maggio JE (1995) 1H NMR of a beta amyloid peptide congeners in water solution. Conformational changes correlate with plaque competence. Biochemistry 34:5191–5200.

Lemere CA, Maron R, Selkoe DJ, Weiner HL. (2001) Nasal vaccination with β-amyloid peptide for the treatment of Alzheimer's disease. DNA Cell Biol 20: 705–711

Lorenzo A, Yankner BA. (1994) β-Amyloid neurotoxicity requires fibril formation and is inhibited by Congo red. Proc Natl Acad Sci USA 91:12243–12247

Maggio JE, Mantyh PW (1996) Brain β-amyloid – a physicochemical perspective. Brain Pathol 6:147–162

Moechars D, Lorent K, De Strooper B, Dewachter I, Van Leuven F (1996) Expression in brain of amyloid precursor protein mutated in the alpha-secretase site causes disturbed behavior, neuronal degeneration and premature death in transgenic mice. EMBO J 15:1265–1274

Naslund J, Haroutunian V, Mohs R, Davis KL Davies P, Greengard P, Buxbaum JD (2000) Correlation between elevated levels of amyloid beta-peptide in the brain and cognitive decline. JAMA 83:1615-1617

Pike CJ, Overman MJ, Cotman CW (1995) Amino-terminal deletions enhance aggregation of β-amyloid peptides *in vitro*. J Biol Chem 270:23895–23898

Schenk D, Barbour R, Dunn W, Gordon G, Grajeda H, Guido T, Hu K, Huang J, Johnson-Wood K, Khan K, Kholodenko D, Lee M, Zhenmei L, Lieberburg I, Motter R, Mutter L, Soriano F, Shopp G, Vasquez N, Vandevert C, Walker S, Wogulis M, Yednock T, Games D, Seubert P (1999) Immunization with amyloid-β attenuates Alzheimer's disease-like pathology in the PDAPP mouse. Nature 400: 173–177

Sigurdsson EM, Scholtzova H, Mehta PD, Frangione B, Wisniewski T (2001) Immunization with a nontoxic/nonfibrillar amyloid-beta homologous peptide reduces Alzheimer's disease-associated pathology in transgenic mice. Am J Pathol 159:439–447

Small DH, Mok SS, Bornstein JC (2001) Alzheimer's disease and A-beta toxicity: from top to bottom. Nature Rev Neurosci 2:595–598

Solomon B (2001) Imunotherapeutic strategies towards prevention and treatment of Alzheimer's disease. DNA Cell Biol 20:697–703

Solomon B, Balas N (1991) Thermostabilization of carboxypeptidase A by interaction with its monoclonal antibodies. Biotechnol Appl Biochem 14:202–211

Solomon B, Frenkel D (2000) Vaccination for the prevention and treatment of Alzheimer's disease. Drugs Today 36:655–663

Solomon B, Schwartz F (1995) Chaperone-like effect of monoclonal antibodies on refolding of heat-denatured carboxypeptidase A.J Mol Recognit 8:72–76

Solomon B, Koppel R, Hanan E, Katzav T (1996) Monoclonal antibodies inhibit *in vitro* fibrillar aggregation of the Alzheimer beta-amyloid peptide. Proc Natl Acad Sci USA 9:452–455.

Solomon B, Koppel R, Frankel D, Hanan-Aharon E. (1997) Disaggregation of Alzheimer β-amyloid by site-directed mAβ. Proc Natl Acad Sci USA 94:4109–4112

Soto C (1999) Plaque busters: strategies to inhibit amyloid formation in Alzheimer's disease. Mol Med Today 5:343–350

Soto C, Castano EM, Frangione B, Inestrosa NC (1995). The α-helical to β-strand transition in the amino-terminal fragment of the amyloid β-peptide modulates amyloid formation. J Biol Chem 270:3063–3067

Talafous J, Marcinowski KJ, Klopman G, Zagorski MG (1994) Solution structure of residues 1-28 of the amyloid beta-peptide. Biochemistry 33:7788–7796

Van Leuven F (2000) Single and multiple transgenic mice as models for Alzheimer's disease. Prog Neurobiol 61: 305–312

Wetzel R (1994) Mutations and off-pathway aggregation of proteins. Trends Biotechnol 12: 193–198

Wisniewski T, Castano EM, Golabek A, Vogel T, Frangione B (1994) Acceleration of Alzheimer's fibril formation by apolipoprotein E *in vitro*. Am J Pathol 145:1030–1035

Characterization of Amyloid Beta Vaccination Strategies in Mice

C. Cao[1], K. E. Ugen[1]*, C. Dickey[2], D. Wilcock[2], Y. Bai[1], M. N. Gordon[2] and D. Morgan[2]

Summary

A beta amyloid (Aβ) peptide vaccine can decrease brain Aβ deposition as well as partially protect against memory loss in a transgenic mouse model for Alzheimer's Disease (AD) that expresses human amyloid precursor protein (APP) and presenilin-1 (PS-1). Current information indicates that antibodies elicited by this vaccine probably mediate the protective effect, although the precise mechanism of action for these antibodies has not yet been established. One of our major interests has been the more extensive characterization of the Aβ vaccine, as well as developing methods for optimizing and maximizing this vaccine strategy. Optimization is important since we have observed that at least three vaccinations with the Aβ peptide vaccine were needed to elicit a significant antibody response. Also, a less robust antibody response to the Aβ vaccine was noted in older animals (i.e., 23 months of age) than in younger animals (4 and 15 months of age).

We have also generated a number of Aβ peptides through recombinant DNA technology and have used some of these to produce vaccines in mice and compared their immunogenicity to Aβ generated by conventional peptide synthetic technology. Vaccination with recombinant Aβ was able to induce significant anti-Aβ antibody levels after only a single immunization, whereas three vaccinations with the Aβ peptide were needed to attain a similar antibody titer. In addition, endpoint anti-Aβ antibody titers were higher after recombinant Aβ vaccination than with peptide Aβ ((approximately 260,000 versus 65,000). These results indicate that the recombinant Aβ may have better efficacy as a vaccine. At present the non-fibrillar/fibrillar nature of the recombinant Aβ preparation is unclear. Work is ongoing to determine the nature of this preparation.

[1] Dept. of Medical Microbiology and Immunology

[2] Alzheimer Research Laboratory, Department of Pharmacology, University of South Florida College of Medicine, Tampa, FL 33612

* Corresponding Author: Kenneth E. Ugen, Ph.D., Dept. of Medical Microbiology and Immunology, University of South Florida College of Medicine, MDC 10, 12901 Bruce B. Downs Boulevard, Tampa, FL 33612, Phone: 813-974-1917, FAX: 813-974-0772, email: kugen@hsc.usf.edu

Selkoe/Christen
Immunization Against Alzheimer's Disease and Other Neurodegenerative Disorders
© Springer-Verlag Berlin Heidelberg 2003

Introduction

Alzheimer's Disease (AD) is a devastating neurodegenerative disease that currently affects approximately four million people in the US. As the baby boomer population ages, this number is expected to increase to nearly 10 million or more in the coming decades. Such an increase in new cases of this devastating disorder will put new and tremendous burdens on the health care system of the US. These dire statistics underscore the necessity for the development of novel preventative and therapeutic approaches against AD.

Progress in AD research has benefited significantly from the development of transgenic murine models, that overexpress APP (Games et al. 1995; Hsiao et al. 1996; Hsiao 1998; Sturchler-Pierrat et al. 1997). This development is particularly important since monitoring the effects of therapeutic interventions on the immunopathological manifestations of AD can only be performed in an animal model, as they can only be measured at necropsy. This fact eliminates the possibility of using human subjects for these types of analyses. Currently, there are several lines of transgenic mice that overexpress mutated forms of human APP. These murine models gradually accumulate $A\beta$ deposits, which become mainly localized in the hippocampus as well as in the cerebral cortex. Cross breeding of APP lines with mice expressing PS-1 accelerates most of the steps in the development of most of the pathology and has provided a useful model for studying AD (Duff et al. 1996). This has led to the hypothesis that the cause of AD centers around Ab (Hardy and Allsop 1991; Hardy 1997).

In vitro aggregation of $A\beta$ likely precipitates a chronic and deleterious process in the brain. It has been shown that activation of both microglia and astrocytes occurs in the vicinity of senile plaques in the brains of AD patients. APP synthesis is apparently regulated by interleukin, such as IL-1, whereby the amyloid plaques stimulate microglial activation and cytokine production. This stimulation could then result in even greater levels of APP.

From a prophylactic and therapeutic standpoint, there has been essentially nothing that could be done to decrease the deposition of $A\beta$ in transgenic mice. In 1999 Schenk and colleagues reported that vaccinating the PDAPP Tg mouse strain (with a transgene that is under the control of a platelet-derived growth factor promoter) with an $A\beta1-42$ peptide, a component of APP, either prevented or significantly decreased $A\beta$ deposits in the cerebral cortex. Also, in these vaccinated animals, activated microglial were found in the hippocampus of 18-month-old mice in association with $A\beta$, suggesting at least some degree of inflammation. Subsequent to this study, the same group under the direction of Bard (Bard et al. 2000) demonstrated that the effect of vaccination on $A\beta$ deposits could apparently be mediated by humoral immunity, as indicated by the use of pooled anti-Ab antisera and murine monoclonal antibodies.

Subsequently, Weiner et al. (2000) showed that nasal administration of the $A\beta$ peptide decreases cerebral amyloid burden in a PDAPP transgenic mouse model for AD. They found that the decrease in $A\beta$ burden was associated with decreased local microglial and astrocyte activation as well as the development of $A\beta$ antibodies of the IgG1 and IgG2b classes, indicating the importance of type II T helper cell responses. In addition, they demonstrated that mononuclear cells in the brain of Aβ mucosally vaccinated animals expressed anti-inflammatory cytokines IL-4, IL-10 and TGF-a (Weiner et al., 2000).

Further studies by Bacskai et al. (2001) demonstrated through multi-photon imaging that local application of Aβ antibody to brains of live PDAPP mice resulted in clearance of cerebral Aβ plaques. Other important work in the area of immune responses against Aβ has been done in Beka Solomon's group in Tel Aviv. Her lab (Frenkelet al. 2000a,b) showed that vaccination of mice with an engineered filamentous phage that expresses the Ab 3-6 epitope (EFRH) resulted in anti-Aβ antibodies of significant titer. Previously, Solomon's lab demonstrated that monoclonal antibodies that recognize the amino region of Aβ could prevent the formation of Aβ fibrils (Solomon et al. 1996) and cause disaggregation of preformed Aβ fibrils (Solomon et al. 1997).

Most recently we (Morgan et al. 2000) as well as others (Janus et al. 2000) have demonstrated that vaccination of APP + PS-1 Tg mice for AD can protect them from behavioral deficits that normally occur in these mice; these behavioral deficits are somewhat analogous to those occurring in human AD patients. This effect was accompanied by a modest decrease in the level of cerebral Aβ in the vaccinated mice.

One working hypothesis for the ability of Aβ peptide vaccination to decrease Aβ deposits is Fc-mediated phagocytosis. One piece of evidence supporting this hypothesis is that microglia are co-localized with Aβ peptide within plaques using confocal microscopy techniques. Also, and importantly, microglia/monocytes, as detected by the presence of MHC complex II-positive staining, were found almost exclusively near the few remaining plaques, as reported by Schenk et al. (1999). However, recently other hypotheses have been put forward to explain the mechanism of action of the Aβ vaccine. One such hypothesis is based on the interesting and important finding by DeMattos et al. (2001) that suggests that the beneficial effects of the antibodies induced by the Aβ vaccine in mice may be mediated by sequestering plasma Aβ, resulting in the movement of at least some of cerebral Aβ down its concentration gradient into the plasma.

Mounting evidence has indicated that Aβ deposition plays a central role in the development of AD (Suh 1997). Importantly, as indicated above, vaccination of mice transgenic for APP and PS-1 with Aβ decreases the pathology in these mice and protects them from associated memory deficits (Morgan et al. 2000). In our hands the Aβ peptide vaccine requires three vaccinations to yield significant anti-Aβ antibody titers and up to nine are required to elicit a half-maximal antibody titer in excess of 10,000. While it is unclear what antibody titer is required to lead to the protective effects of this vaccine in mice, it will be important to develop other Aβ reagents that will more effectively and efficiently induce high antibody titers. This report summarizes our efforts to develop such reagents.

It has been reported that the synthetic Aβ peptide can undergo different conformations while being reconstituted (Podlisny et al. 1998; Huang et al. 2000). In addition, the role of fibrillar aggregates of Aβ in the etiology and pathogenesis of AD has not yet been firmly established. We recently addressed the question of the ability of different preparations of recombinant Aβ (rAβ) to elicit humoral immune responses. Specifically, we cloned the Aβ into an expression vector (pGEX-6p-1) that carries the GST gene. The rationale for making these recombinant proteins was that these preparations may more directly mimic biologically relevant forms (in terms of peptide/protein conformation) than does the Aβ produced by conventional peptide synthetic technology.

Materials and Methods

Antibody Responses to Ab 1-42 Peptide (pAβ) Vaccination

The methods for the preparation of the Aβ 1-42 peptide for vaccination have been described in previously published studies (Morgan et al. 2000; Dickey et al. 2001; Wilcock et al. 2001). Briefly, for the initial vaccination studies reported in papers, the Aβ peptide was prepared so as to probably result in an aggregated/fibrillar preparation. The peptide was then emulsified in Freund's adjuvant for vaccination. Mice were vaccinated with 100 μg of peptide of peptide Aβ 1-42 at 2, 2.5, 3.5, 4.5, 5.5, 6.5, 7.5, 8.5 and 9.5 months of age. Bleeds were taken to determine anti-Aβ antibodies at 2, 3, 4, 5, 6, 7, 8, 9, 10, 14, 18 and 24 months. Immobilzed Aβ was used at a concentration of 5 μg/ml with 250 ng added per well. Mean half-maximal antibody titers were calculated based on binding of antisera to immobilized peptide Aβ 1-42 by ELISA.

Cloning Strategy for Aβ 1-42 DNA

The DNA sequence of the first 42 amino acids of Aβ was obtained from the NCBI Genbank database. The following oligonucleotides were designed to amplify the human Aβ 1-42 gene:

p1 (Sense)   5'--- gatgcagaat tccgacatga ctcaggatat gaagttcatc
                      atcaaaaatt ggtgttcttt gcagaagatgtgggg---3'

p2 (Antisense) 5'-- cgc tatgacaaca ccgcccacca tgagtccaat
                     gattgcacct ttgtttgaac ccacatcttc tgcaaagaac acca--3'
p3 (Sense)   5'---gccgccggatccatggatgcagaat tccgacatga---3'
p4 (Antisense)   5'--gccgccgacatcttacgc tatgacaaca ccgccca---3'

p1 and P2 were annealed to obtain the full length Aβ gene. The gene was then amplified by PCR. The *Bam*HI and *Eco*RV restriction sites were then added by PCR, using primers P3 and P4. The resulting amplicons were cloned into TOPO-TA2.1 vectors and positive clones were selected.

Expression of Recombinant Aβ Proteins

The Aβ 1-42 gene was cloned into a TA vector and then sub-cloned into pGEX-6p-1 (a GST fusion vector) to make pGEX-6p-1/Aβ. pGEX-6p-1/Aβ was then transformed into BL21 host bacteria. Recombinant GST-Aβ protein was expressed in BL21 under induction by 0.1 mM IPTG. Bacteria were sonicated and the recombinant GST-Aβ was isolated on a Sepharose 4B column. Beads binding the GST-Aβ were digested by PreScission Protease to release rAβ. The recombinant proteins were purified and confirmed as Aβ 1-42 through electrophoresis and Western blotting using a commercially obtained anti-Aβ monoclonal antibody (data not shown).

Reactivity of a Commercial Monoclonal Antibody Against rAβ and pAβ

A comparison was made between the binding of a commercial anti-Aβ murine monoclonal antibody (purchased from Chemicon International Inc. with a specificity for amino acids 1-16) to rAβ and pAβ. This comparison was performed to determine whether the recombinant Aβ generated in this report could be recognized by antibodies generated against Aβ produced by synthetic peptide methods.

Binding of Pooled Sera from pAβ Vaccinated Mice to rAβ

A pool of sera from mice vaccinated nine times (n = 5) with pAβ was used in an ELISA at a range of dilutions to determine the ability of these sera to recognize recombinant Aβ.

rAβ Vaccination of Transgenic (Tg) Mice

Fifty μg/100μl of the recombinant Aβ protein prepared as described above was used as an immunogen in transgenic mice. Briefly the rAβ was mixed with 100 μl complete Freund's adjuvant (CFA) and was emulsified completely by syringe and then subcutaneously injected into Tg mice. Mice were boosted with 50 μg of rAβ two times at two-week intervals and were bled two weeks after the third injection. ELISA were performed to test the ability of the antisera from these vaccinated mice to recognize rAβ and peptide Aβ. In addition the antibody titers were compared to a pool of antisera from transgenic mice (n = 5) that had been vaccinated nine times with the peptide Aβ vaccine.

Anti-Aβ 1Antibody Titers as a Function of Mouse Age at Time of Vaccination

Four-, 15- and 23-month-old PS-1 mice (five from each group) were vaccinated four times with 100 μg of peptide Aβ 1-42 (pAβ) at two-week intervals. Blood was taken two weeks after the final vaccination to determine the anti-Aβ 1-42 antibody titer. This experiment was performed to determine whether there is differential efficiency in eliciting anti-Aβ antibody titers in mice as a function of age at vaccination.

Results and Discussion

We have demonstrated that a nine-vaccination regimen similar to the one utilized by Schenk et al. can result in at least partial protection against memory deficits in doubly transgenic APP + PS-1 mice (Morgan et al. 2000). Such an effect, as indicated above, has been documented independently by another group using a similar transgenic mouse model (Janus et al. 2000). Although a sizable anti-Aβ antibody titer was attained after this vaccination scheme, it was noted that at least three vaccinations were needed to attain a measurable anti-Aβ titer.

Logistically, it is more favorable for vaccines to elicit a protective immune response with as few vaccinations as possible. We therefore decided to develop different Aβ preparations using recombinant DNA technology. These preparations can then be used as vaccines and questions on improved immunogenicity and efficacy can then be addressed.

Figure 1 shows the time course of antibody responses in transgenic mice vaccinated with commercial Aβ 1-42 peptide (Bachem, Inc). The initial vaccination (100 μg) was made in two-month-old mice, followed by vaccinations at approximately one-month intervals up until 9.5 months of age. Anti-Aβ titers were determined at one-month intervals from 2 through 24 months. Only after three vaccinations did we attain antibody titers in excess of 40. The antibody titers steadily increased with each successive vaccination and slowly declined after the final vaccination. Importantly, the anti-Aβ antibody titer was still approximately 5,000 at nine months after the final vaccination and declined to 2,000 at 15 months after the final vaccination. It was unclear what antibody titer level needed to be attained and maintained to mediate a protective effect, either in terms of decreasing cerebral amyloid load or protecting from memory deficits.

Therefore, it was decided to generate Aβ 1-42 through recombinant DNA technology. The cloning strategy for generating these reagents is summarized in the Materials and Methods section. In summary, the Aβ recombinant protein was generated by overlapping PCR and cloned into the pGEX-6p-1 vector and then expressed. Using glutathione Sepharose 4B, the purified, bound GST fusion protein (rAβ-GST) was cut from GST by enzyme digestion.

The identity of the rAβ generated by this method was confirmed through Western blotting analysis. The rAβ preparation was further characterized by ELISA using a commercial anti-Aβ murine monoclonal antibody (AβMab) with specificity for the first 16 amino acids. At a range of dilutions of the AβMab from

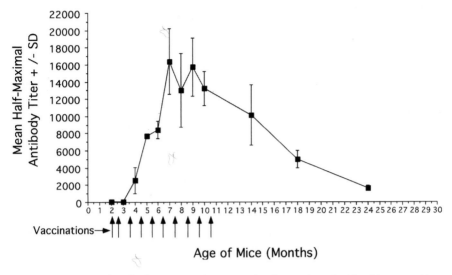

Fig. 1. Time course of antibody responses in transgenic mice vaccinated with Aβ 1-42 peptide

1:500 through 1:6000, the rAβ exhibited consistently higher binding to the AβMab than did pAβ (Fig. 2A). In addition, a pool of antisera from pAβ vaccinated mice was as effective in binding to rAβ at a wide range of dilutions as it was in binding to pAβ (Fig. 2B).

When rAβ was used as a vaccine in transgenic mice it was able to elicit antibodies with greater binding affinity to pAβ by ELISA than did the pool of antisera from pAβ-vaccinated mice (Fig. 3). In this experiment the end-point antibody titer of pooled antisera from pAβ-vaccinated mice against pAβ was 65,536. Conversely, the end-point titer from rAβ-vaccinated mice against pAβ was greater than 262,144 but less than 1,048,576. Importantly, the pool of antisera from the pAβ-vaccinated mice was collected after nine vaccinations whereas the pool from the rAβ–vaccinated mice was collected after only three vaccinations. These results indicate that not only did the rAβ elicit specific anti-Aβ antibodies of higher titer than did pAβ but also that it resulted in the generation of these titer levels with far fewer vaccinations.

An additional important area to consider when devising vaccines for use in the aged, such as a potential AD vaccine, is the likely influence of immunosenescence on vaccination efficacy. It has been indicated that both humoral and cellular immunosenescense occurs with aging (Miller 1995). To test this hypothesis we decided to vaccinate four-, 15- and 23-month-old mice (five from each group) four times with 100 μg of peptide Aβ 1-42 (pAβ) at two-week intervals. Sera were then collected two weeks after the final vaccination to determine the anti-Aβ 1-42 antibody titer. The data from these experiments are presented in Figure 4. As expected, after two vaccinations a measurable anti Aβ antibody titer was not at-

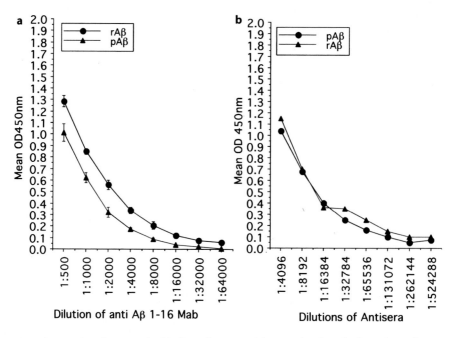

Fig. 2. Comparison between the binding of commercial monoclonal antibody against Aβ 1-22 peptide (pAβ) and recombinant Aβ 1-42 (rAβ)

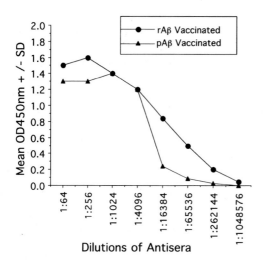

Fig. 3. Antibody titer after vaccination by rAβ and pAβ.

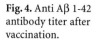

Fig. 4. Anti Aβ 1-42 antibody titer after vaccination.

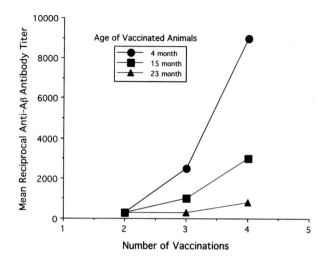

tained in any of the age groups. After three and four vaccinations, substantial antibody titers were attained in the young (four-month) age group while considerably lower titers were measured in the middle age group (15 months) and less still in the oldest age group (23 months). These data indicate that efficacy problems in terms of mounting a substantial humoral immune response might be encountered with an Aβ vaccine targeted to the aged. This finding underscores the importance of developing methods for enhancing immune responses in this population. This problem could be addressed through the development of novel adjuvant approaches, including the co-delivery of immunomodulatory cytokines that could drive Th2 immune responses that are important for the development of humoral immunity.

In summary, we report in this paper the generation of an Aβ 1-42 molecule by recombinant DNA technology which appears to have some advantages, in terms of immunogenicity, over the peptide. Further analysis of this preparation in mouse model systems is ongoing. At present, it is unclear what the fibrillar nature of our rAβ preparation is, so work to determine the nature of this preparation is also ongoing.

Acknowledgments

This work was supported in part by grants from the National Institute on Aging of the NIH to K. Ugen (AG20227) and D. Morgan (AG18478).

References

Bacskai J, Kajdasz ST, Christie RH, Carter C, Games D, Seubert P, Schenk D, Hyman BT (2001) Imaging of amyloid-beta deposits in brains of living mice permits direct observation of clearance of plaques with immunotherapy. Nature Med 7:369–372.

Bard F, Cannon C, Barbour R, Burke RL, Games D, Grajeda H, Guido T, Hu K, Huang J, Johnson-Wood K, Khan K, Kholodenko D, Lee M, Lieberburg I, Motter R, Nguyen M, Soriano F, Vasquez N, Weiss K, Welch B, Seubert P, Schenk D, Yednock T (2000) Peripherally administered antibodies against amyloid beta-peptide enter the central nervous system and reduce pathology in a mouse model of Alzheimer disease. Nature Med 6:916–919.

DeMattos RB, Bales KR, Cummins DJ, Dodart JC, Paul SM, Holtzman DM (2001) Peripheral anti-A beta antibody alters CNS and plasma A beta clearance and decreases brain A beta burden in a mouse model of Alzheimer's disease. Proc Natl Acad Sci USA 98:8850–8855.

Dickey CA, Morgan DG, Kudchodkar S, Weiner DB, Bai Y, Cao C, Gordon MN, Ugen KE (2001) Duration and specificity of humoral immune responses in mice vaccinated with the Alzheimer's disease-associated beta-amyloid 1-42 peptide. DNA Cell Biol 20:723–729.

Duff K, Eckman C, Zehr C, Yu X, Prada CM, Perez-tur J, Hutton M, Buee L, Harigaya Y, Yager D, Morgan D, Gordon M, Holcomb L, Refolo L, Zenk B, Hardy J, Younkin S (1996) Increased amyloid-beta42(43) in brains of mice expressing mutant presenilin 1. Nature 383:710–713.

Frenkel D, Katz O, Solomon B (2000a) Immunization against Alzheimer's beta -amyloid plaques via EFRH phage administration. Proc Natl Acad Sci USA 97:11455–11459.

Frenkel D, Solomon B, Benhar I (2000b) Modulation of Alzheimer's beta-amyloid neurotoxicity by site-directed single-chain antibody. J Neuroimmunol 106:23–31.

Games D, Adams D, Alessandrini R, Barbour R, Berthelette P, Blackwell C, Carr T, Clemens J, Donaldson T, Gillespie F, Guido T, Hagopian S, Johnson-Wood K, Khan K, Lee M, Leibowitz P, Lieberburg I, Little S, Masliah E, McConlogue L, Montoya-Zavala M, Mucke L, Paganini L, Penniman E, Power M, Schenk D, Seubert P, Snyder B, Soriano F, Tan H, Vitale J, Wadsworth S, Wolozin B, Zhao J (1995) Alzheimer-type neuropathology in transgenic mice overexpressing V717F beta-amyloid precursor protein. Nature 373:523–527

Hardy J (1997) Amyloid, the presenilins and Alzheimer's disease. Trends Neurosci 20:154–159.

Hardy J, Allsop D (1991). Amyloid deposition as the central event in the aetiology of Alzheimer's disease. Trends Pharmacol Sci 12:383–388.

Hsiao K (1998) Strain dependent and invariant features of transgenic mice expressing Alzheimer amyloid precursor proteins. Prog Brain Res 117:335–341.

Hsiao K, Chapman P, Nilsen S, Eckman C, Harigaya Y, Younkin S, Yang F, Cole G (1996) Correlative memory deficits, Aβ elevation, and amyloid plaques in transgenic mice. Science 274:99–102.

Huang T H, Yang DS, Plaskos NP, Go S, Yip CM, Fraser PE, Chakrabartty A (2000) Structural studies of soluble oligomers of the Alzheimer beta-amyloid peptide. J Mol Biol 297:73–87.

Janus C, Pearson J, McLaurin, J, Mathews PM, Jiang Y, Schmidt SD, Chishti MA, Horne P, Heslin D, French J, Mount HT, Nixon RA, Mercken M, Bergeron C, Fraser PE, St George-Hyslop P, Westaway D (2000) A beta peptide immunization reduces behavioural impairment and plaques in a model of Alzheimer's disease. Nature 408:979–982.

Miller RA (1995) Immune systems. In: Masoro E (ed) Handbook of physiology. Section 11: Physiology of aging. New York: Oxford University Press, pp 555–590.

Morgan D, Diamond DM, Gottschall PE, Ugen KE, Dickey C, Hardy,J, Duff K, Jantzen P, DiCarlo G, Wilcock D, Connor K, Hatcher J, Hope C, Gordon M, Arendash GW (2000) A beta peptide vaccination prevents memory loss in an animal model of Alzheimer's disease. Nature 408:982–985.

Podlisny MB, Walsh DM, Amarante P, Ostaszewski BL, Stimson ER, Maggio JE, Teplow DB, Selkoe DJ (1998) Oligomerization of endogenous and synthetic amyloid beta-protein at nanomolar levels in cell culture and stabilization of monomer by Congo red. Biochemistry 37:3602–3611.

Schenk D, Barbour R, Dunn W, Gordon G, Grajeda H, Guido T, Hu K, Huang J, Johnson-Wood K, Khan K, Kholodenko D, Lee M, Liao Z, Lieberburg I, Motter R, Mutter L, Soriano F, Shopp G, Vasquez N, Vandevert C, Walker S, Wogulis M, Yednock T, Games D, Seubert P (1999) Immunization with amyloid-beta attenuates Alzheimer-disease-like pathology in the PDAPP mouse. Nature 400:173–177.

Solomon B, Koppel R, Hanan E, Katzav T (1996) Monoclonal antibodies inhibit in vitro fibrillar aggregation of the Alzheimer beta-amyloid peptide. Proc Natl Acad Sci USA 93:452–455.

Solomon B, Koppel R, Frankel D, Hanan-Aharon E (1997) Disaggregation of Alzheimer beta-amyloid by site-directed mAb. Proc Natl Acad Sci USA 94:4109–4112.

Sturchler-Pierrat C, Abramowski D, Duke M, Wiederhold KH, Mistl C, Rothacher S, Ledermann B, Burki K, Frey P, Paganetti PA, Waridel C, Calhoun ME, Jucker M, Probst A, Staufenbiel M, Sommer B (1997) Two amyloid precursor protein transgenic mouse models with Alzheimer disease-like pathology. Proc Natl Acad Sci USA 94:13287–13292.

Suh YH (1997). An etiological role of amyloidogenic carboxyl-terminal fragments of the beta-amyloid precursor protein in Alzheimer's disease. J Neurochem 68:1781–1791.

Weiner HL, Lemere CA, Maron, R, Spooner ET, Grenfell, TJ, Mori C, Issazadeh S, Hancock WW, Selkoe DJ (2000) Nasal administration of amyloid-beta peptide decreases cerebral amyloid burden in a mouse model of Alzheimer's disease. Ann Neurol 48:567–579.

Wilcock DM, Gordon MN, Ugen KE, Gottschall PE, DiCarlo G, Dickey C, Boyett KW, Jantzen PT, Connor KE, Melachrino J, Hardy J, Morgan D (2001) Number of Abeta inoculations in APP+PS1 transgenic mice influences antibody titers, microglial activation, and congophilic plaque levels. DNA Cell Biol 20:731–736.

Cognitive Characteristics of TgAPP CRND8 Mice Immunised with Beta Amyloid Peptide

C. Janus, H.-S. Johnson, J. McLaurin, P. Fraser, P. St. George-Hyslop and D. Westaway[1]

The progressive cognitive dysfunction of Alzheimer's disease (AD) is accompanied by a series of neuropathological changes, including deposition of amyloid β peptide in the parenchyma and blood vessels (Aβ) of the human brain. Many lines of evidence indicate that abnormal processing of Aβ (a proteolytic derivative of the β-amyloid precursor protein – βAPP) plays a central role in initiating the pathogenesis of AD (reviewed in Steineret al. 1999). There are also data indicating a positive correlation between β-amyloid plaques and cognitive impairment in AD patients (Cummings et al.1996; Haroutunian et al. 1998; Kanne et al.1998). However, there are gaps in our knowledge of the pathogenesis of even the "simple" genetic forms of AD. Thus there has been a need for an animal model that develops some or all aspects of this uniquely human disease in a reproducible fashion to decipher and stratify crucial pathogenic events. Such animal models would also, of course, be useful for testing therapies.

Current transgenic mouse models of AD fall short of recapitulating all the pathological changes seen in this disease, or have confounding neuroanatomical perturbations, or have rather evanescent behavioural phenotypes. Nonetheless, some Tg models of AD, such as the Tg PDAPP mice, do develop incontrovertible AD-like, mature amyloid deposits and researchers have used these to venture into "second-generation" experiments to assess candidate therapies. One recent breakthrough in this field investigated the use of immunization against the Aβ peptide. These studies documented significant reduction in the β-amyloid plaque burden in the Tg PDAPP mouse brain (Schenk et al. 1999). A follow-up report proved that antibodies against amyloid-β peptide, when given peripherally to mice via passive administration, were sufficient to reduce amyloid burden via induction of clearance of pre-existing amyloid (Bard et al. 2000). In addition to pioneering a particular therapeutic regimen, these studies were important in that they established that AD amyloid deposits, long-regarded as insoluble and metabolically inert, are in fact labile, as now confirmed by the use of other experimental paradigms (Nakagawa et al. 2000). However, the effect of immunisation with Aβ peptide on learning and memory in a mouse Tg model was not addressed in the above studies. Evidence that Aβ immunisation also reduces cognitive dysfunction in murine models of AD would strongly support the hypothesis that abnormal Aβ processing is critical to the pathogenesis of AD and would encourage

---

[1] Centre for Research in Neurodegenerative Disease. University of Toronto, 6 Queen's Park Crescent West, Toronto, Ontario M9B 5K3, Canada

Selkoe/Christen
Immunization Against Alzheimer's Disease
and Other Neurodegenerative Disorders
© Springer-Verlag Berlin Heidelberg 2003

the development of strategies directed at intervening at various points in the "amyloid cascade" (Steiner et al. 1999).

The experiment evaluating the effect of Aβ immunisation on cognition in a transgenic mouse model has to incorporate longitudinal administration of an immunogen (Schenk et al. 1999), and the behavioural paradigm should take into account the following characteristics of behavioural deficits in AD patients. First, in AD there are defects in multiple spheres of cognitive function (several types of memory, judgement, executive planning, motor praxias, cognitive processing speed, etc.). Thus, AD is not just a disease of learning or of memory (Katzman et al. 1999). Secondly, learning is not completely absent in AD patients until very late in the disease, when there has been massive cell loss and the patients are bedridden. To replicate this situation, a potential animal model should therefore show slower rate of learning but not its complete absence. Thirdly, the experimental design should mimic designs used in human clinical trial designs and should follow longitudinal administration of the immunogen.

Since the main purpose of the present behavioural experiment was to test the hypothesis that immunisation with the Aβ42 peptide alleviates the cognitive impairment in transgenic APP mice, a longitudinal design was chosen to provide a detailed, overall characterization of alterations in cognitive performance in the same mice during an overall immunisation regimen. The choice of the design followed the premise that it is unlikely that AD patients should ever be treated continuously but evaluated only once. Moreover, and in contrast to cross-sectional, one time-point designs, the longitudinal design exposes the study to the type of confounds likely to be encountered in the real world of clinical trials. These confounds include: potential loss of power due to interference by intercurrent death, re-test [carrying over (Martin and Bateson 1996)] effects, and the reality that the untreated phenotype progresses with time.

We have created a line of transgenic mice, denoted TgCRND8, encoding a compound mutant form of the human amyloid precursor protein, βAPP_{695}, (K670N/M671L and V717F in *cis*) under the regulation of the Syrian Hamster prion promoter on a C3H/B6 strain background (Chishti et al. 2001). By ~12 weeks of age, these mice show significant spatial learning deficits (Fig. 1) that are accompanied by increasing numbers of cortical, Aβ-containing amyloid plaques and by increasing levels of SDS soluble Aβ (Chishti et al. 2001).

To assess the effect of $A\beta_{42}$ immunization on the learning deficits of TgCRND8 mice, age- and sex-matched cohorts of TgCRND8 mice (n = 21) and of non-Tg littermates (n = 39) were repeatedly vaccinated, following the regimen used by Schenk and co-workers (1999), at 6, 8, 12, 16, and 20 weeks with either $A\beta_{42}$ or islet associated polypeptide (IAPP) peptide. IAPP was selected as the control immunogen because it has similar biophysical β-sheet properties but is associated with a non-CNS amyloidosis. The cognitive behaviour of the mice was repeatedly evaluated in the hidden platform version of the Morris water maze test at 11, 15, 19 and 23 weeks of age. At each age of behavioural testing, mice were trained for five days with four trials per day and the hidden platform was placed in a different quadrant of the pool. The water maze was chosen because it allows evaluation not only of spatial learning and memory but also evaluates locomotor and exploratory abilities of mice, and development of appropriate search strategies for a

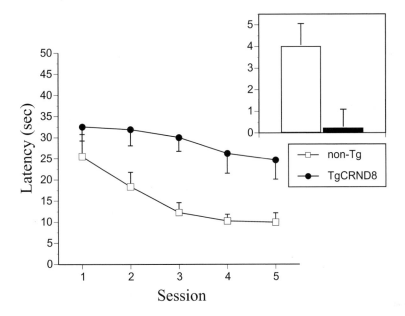

Fig. 1. The TgCRND8 mice show significant impairment in spatial learning and spatial memory (insert) assessed in the water maze test. Experimentally naïve, non-immunised TgCRND8 mice (n = 10) and their non-Tg littermates (n = 7) were trained in the water maze throughout five sessions (days) with four trials per session at 11 weeks of age. Although all mice showed a significant improvement during training, the TgCRND8 mice had significantly longer escape latencies to the hidden platform than non-Tg mice (Genotype × Session interaction was not significant). An insert shows an annulus crossing index during the probe trial administered after learning acquisition phase. The index represents the number of platform site crosses in the target quadrant during the probe trial adjusted for sites crossings in other quadrants (index = TQ -(AR + AL + OP)/3). Highly positive index indicates selective spatial memory for the spatial platform position. TgCRND8 mice showed significant impairment in spatial memory, as assessed by their search for the platform position during the probe trial.

spatial position. Behavioural pilot studies in non-Tg mice established that immunisation with Freund's Adjuvant + phosphate buffered saline, Freund's + $A\beta_{42}$, Freund's + IAPP, IAPP alone, or $A\beta_{42}$ alone all had no specific effect on locomotor performance or perceptual systems of mice in the Morris water maze test. To assess the effect of the vaccination on behaviour, performance in the water maze for the entire 11- to 23-week experimental period was analysed using a mixed model of factorial analysis of variance (ANOVA), with immunogen ($A\beta_{42}$ versus IAPP) and genotype (TgCRND8 versus non-Tg) as between-subject, and age-of-testing (11, 15, 19, 23 weeks) as within-subject, factors.

The main analysis revealed significant immunogen × genotype ($P < 0.01$) and immunogen × genotype × age ($P < 0.05$) interactions, as well as significant main factor effects for immunogen, genotype; age-of-testing ($P < 0.01$ for all)analysis indicated that, although all mice improved their performance during the experiment, the response significantly depended on the type of immunogen and genotype of

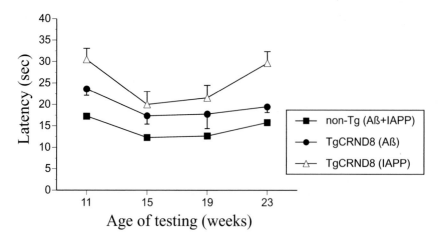

Fig. 2. The overall effect of immunisation with $A\beta_{42}$ peptide on TgCRND8 mice spatial learning during the 11- to – 23 week experimental period. Escape latencies were averaged across all frve sessions of training at each age of longitudinal testing. The performance of $A\beta_{42}$-immunised TgCRND8 mice was similar to that of non-Tg littermates; however, their performance did not reach the level of non-Tg mice. In contrast, IAPP-immunised mice showed longer latencies when compared to $A\beta_{42}$-immunised TgCRND8 mice ($P < 0.05$) and their non-Tg littermates ($Ps < 0.001$).

mice. Consecutive analysis of simple effects revealed that, overall, the $A\beta_{42}$-immunised TgCRND8 mice performed significantly better than IAPP-immunised TgCRND8 mice (immunogen effect within TgCRND8 mice: $P < 0.05$) within the 11- to – 23-week experimental period. Figure 2 shows graphically the age effect as the average escape latency of all five training sessions at each age of testing. The conclusion that $A\beta_{42}$-immunisation ameliorates the cognitive deficit of TgCRND8 mice was robust, regardless of whether the analysis assessed latency to reach the hidden platform or swim path length (a measure less sensitive to swim speed and floating). Furthermore, $A\beta_{42}$ immunisation had a relatively large effect, because 31% of the

---►

Fig. 3. Water maze test performance of TgCRND8 mice at each age of testing. At 11 weeks of age, IAPP-immunised TgCRND8 mice ($n = 12$) show cognitive impairment relative to non-Tg controls ($n = 8$; **a, left**), whereas the performance of $A\beta_{42}$-immunised TgCRND8 mice ($n = 9$; **a, right**) approaches that of non-Tg littermates ($n = 19$). At 15 weeks of age, the IAPP-immunised TgCRND8 mice ($n = 6$; **b, left**) showed significant ($P < 0.01$, $\omega^2 = 36\%$) impairment compared to non-Tg littermates ($n = 16$) but were not different from the $A\beta_{42}$-immunised TgCRND8 mice ($n = 7$; **b, right**). At 19 weeks of age, the IAPP-immunised TgCRND8 mice ($n = 6$; **c, left**) also showed significant ($P < 0.01$, $\omega^2 = 34\%$) impairment compared to non-Tg littermates ($n = 15$) but similar performance to $A\beta_{42}$-immunised TgCRND8 mice ($n = 6$; **c, right**). At 23 weeks of age, the IAPP-immunised TgCRND8 mice ($n = 6$; **d, left**) showed significant ($P < 0.001$, $\omega^2 = 65\%$) impairment compared to non-Tg littermates ($n = 15$), but were also significantly impaired relative to $A\beta_{42}$-immunised TgCRND8 mice ($n = 6$; **d, right**) ($P < 0.01$). Vertical bars represent ±SEM.

variance in the performance of immunized TgCRND8 mice was attributable to the effects of the immunogen. However, although $A\beta_{42}$ immunisation improved behaviour in TgCRND8 mice, it did not fully restore it to the level of non-Tg mice (genotype effect within $A\beta_{42}$-immunized mice was significant: $P < 0.01$; Fig. 2).

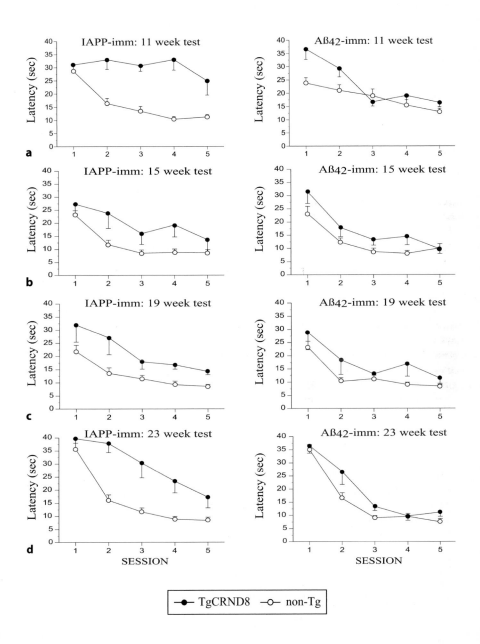

The performance of mice for individual test periods (11, 15, 19 and 23 weeks) is presented in Figure 3. *Post hoc* analyses revealed significant immunogen x genotype interactions at 11 and 23 weeks ($P < 0.02$ and $P < 0.001$, respectively). The subsequent analysis of simple effects revealed that $A\beta_{42}$ immunisation markedly improved spatial learning in TgCRND8 mice relative to IAPP mice at 11 weeks ($P < 0.05$) and 23 weeks ($P < 0.01$). Furthermore, $A\beta_{42}$ immunisation accounted for large portions of the variance in performance at both age periods ($\omega^2 = 19\%$ at 11 weeks; $\omega^2 = 42\%$ at 23 weeks). Analyses at 15 and 19 weeks did not show statistically significant effects. This lack of significant immunisation effect at 15 and 19 weeks, and its reappearance at 23 weeks, may reflect a carring over effect.

In addition to reducing the behavioural deficits, $A\beta_{42}$ immunisation caused significant (~50%) reductions in the number and size of dense-cored plaques containing fibrillar, β-sheet forms of Aβ in the hippocampus and cerebral cortex of TgCRND8 mice (Fig. 4).

A simple explanation of the results is that cerebral amyloid plaques are the toxic moiety and that the modest (~50%) reduction in dense-cored, mature amyloid plaques caused by $A\beta_{42}$ vaccination is sufficient to prevent or reverse the behavioural deficits. However, a more likely alternative explanation is that immunotherapy is active against either a particular conformational species of Aβ (e.g., fibrillar or protofibrillar forms) or Aβ in a restricted compartment. Several lines of evidence favour the former option. First, recent in vitro studies have suggested that small, oligomeric assemblies of Aβ ("protofibrils") are the most neurotoxic conformational species (Hartley et al. 1999; Pike et al.1993; Walsh et al. 1999). Second, these diffusible, toxic forms of Aβ, which comprise only a small proportion of the total Aβ in the brains of AD patients, are the most accurate predictors of neurodegeneration (McLean et al. 1999).

Although producing a strong effect, $A\beta_{42}$ immunisation did not fully reverse the behavioural deficits and neuropathology in TgCRND8 mice. This might reflect either the inefficient ingress of antibodies to the CNS [estimated at 0.1% of serum levels (Bard et al. 2000)] or the fact that other βAPP-proteolytic fragments may also be involved in the pathogenesis of AD (Lu et al. 2000).

Nonetheless, the strong effect of immunisation discerned in this first series of experiments (i.e., without a prior series of experiments to optimize the procedure) speaks to the potential utility of this intervention. Our data imply that either very small reductions in the levels of $A\beta_{42}$ and β-amyloid plaques are sufficient to affect cognition or that vaccination need only modulate the activity/abundance of a small sub-population of toxic fibrillar $A\beta_{42}$ species.

The results obtained in this first experiment (Janus et al. 2000) showed that $A\beta_{42}$ immunisation appeared to be efficacious in younger TgCRND8 mice (the onset of immunization was at six weeks of age, before the amyloid plaque deposition), thus acting in a preventive manner. However, it was not known if such beneficial effect could be observed when older mice, with well-developed pathology, were immunized. We therefore carried out a pilot study (Janus et al. 2001) that confirmed that this was the case in older TgCRND8 mice.

A cohort of TgCRND8 non-immunized mice was longitudinally tested in the reference memory version of a water maze at ages 5, 11, 15, 20, 30, and 40 weeks.

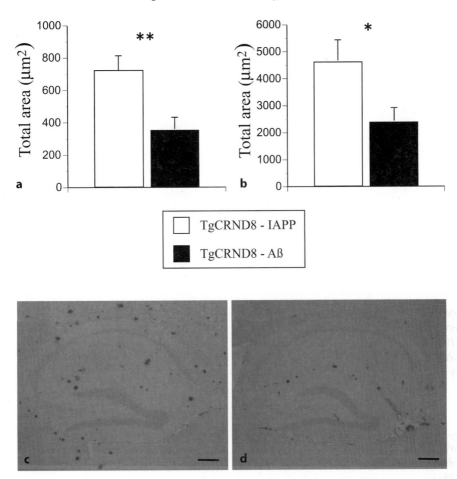

Fig. 4. At the end of experiment (25 weeks of age), the Aβ plaque load of TgCRND8 mice immunised with $A\beta_{42}$ and IAPP peptides was quantified in the hippocampus and in the cerebral cortex. The total area (μm^2) of plaques in Aβ-immunised mice was reduced two-fold, in the hippocampus (**a**, P < 0.01) and in the cortex (**b**, P < 0.05), as compared to Tg mice immunised with control IAPP peptide. Comparison of plaque counts between IAPP- and Aβ-immunised mice yielded a similar two-fold reduction in number of plaques in the hippocampus (20.9 ± 1.7 versus 11.6 ± 1.6 for IAPP- and Aβ-immunised mice, P < 0.01) and in the cortex (119.7 ± 14.6 versus 71.4 ± 10.8 for IAPP- and Aβ-immunised mice, P < 0.05). Representative pictures of the distribution of Aβ plaques in the hippocampal region in IAPP- and $A\beta_{42}$-immunised mice (**c** and **d**, respectively). Vertical bars represent SEM, * P < 0.05, ** P < 0.01. Scale bars represent 100μm.

In early tests, although impaired, the TgCRND8 mice showed a modest reduction in the perceived "impairment" in this experimental paradigm, likely due to a carry-over effect of repeated testing. However, during later tests at ages of 20, 30, and 40 weeks, the Tg mice showed a stable and significant impairment in spatial navigation (Fig. 5).

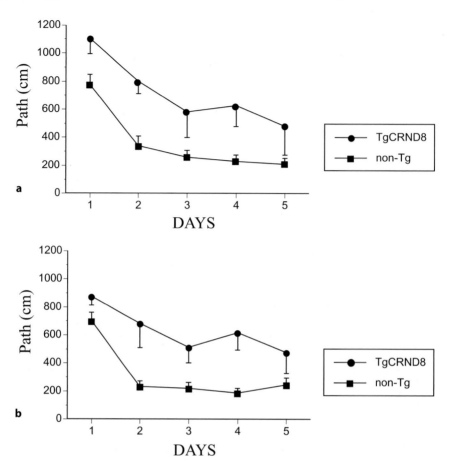

Fig. 5. Compared to their non-Tg littermates, Tg(APP)CRND8 mice take significantly longer to search for the submerged platform during re-tests at 30 weeks (P < 0.01; **a**) and 40 weeks of age (P < 0.01; **b**). The search path is reported since it is relatively unaffected by the floating observed in older mice.

The mice (Tg and non-Tg littermates) were immunised with $A\beta_{42}$ peptide at 46 weeks and their spatial navigation was tested at 51, 55, and 59 weeks of age. The results demonstrated that immunisation of old TgCRND8 mice improved their cognitive performance in the water maze (Fig. 6).

However, the onset of the effect was observed after longer administration of the antigen (four immunizations, 13 weeks after the onset of the experiment) as compared to the previously reported (Janus et al. 2000) "early" immunisation of mice at six weeks (a significant improvement in performance was observed after two immunizations five weeks after the onset of the experiment). These findings are encouraging, but have to be repeated on larger sample sizes of mice to compare the effects of immunization at early and late ages.

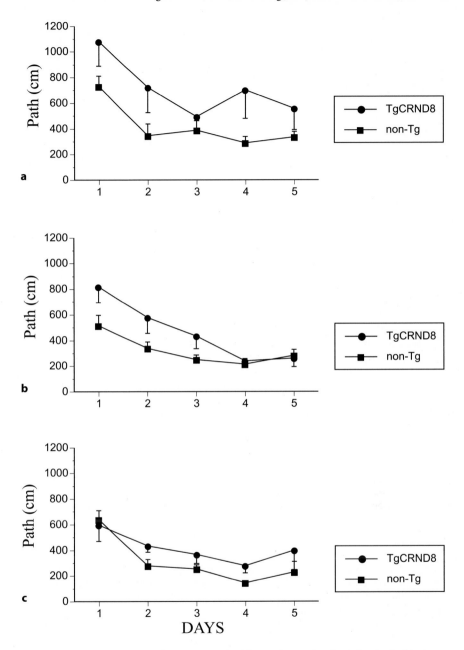

Fig. 6. Impaired in spatial navigation, 45-week-old TgCRND8 mice showed a gradual improvement in search for a submerged platform position in the water maze after immunisation with Aβ42 peptide. The mice still showed an impairment in tests carried out five (**a**; p = 0.03) or nine (**b**; p = 0.05) weeks from the onset of immunisation (age: 51 and 55 weeks, respectively). However, they improved significantly (P > 0.05) during the third re-test after 12 weeks from the beginning of immunisation, showing performance comparable to their non-Tg littermates (**c**).

Overall, these findings in experimental animals have positive implications for further iterations of the immunisation procedure. While these experiments were not designed to address potential side effects that may be encountered at the bedside, they comprise something of a proof-of-principle for several incipient therapies directed against the Aβ amyloid cascade.

References

Bard F, Cannon C, Barbour R, Burke RL, Games D, Grajeda H, Guido T, Hu K, Huang J, Johnson-Wood K, Khan K, Kholodenko D, Lee M, Lieberburg I, Motter R, Nguyen M, Soriano, F, Vasquez N, Weiss K, Welch B, Seubert P, Schenk D, Yednock T (2000) Peripherally administered antibodies against amyloid beta-peptide enter the central nervous system and reduce pathology in a mouse model of Alzheimer disease. Nature Med 6:916–919

Chishti MA, Yang DS, Janus C, Phinney, AL, Horne P, Pearson J, Strome R, Zuker N, Loukides J, French J, Turner S, Lozza G, Grilli, M, Kunicki S, Morissette C, Paquette J, Gervais F, Bergeron C, Fraser, PE, Carlson GA, George-Hyslop PS, Westaway D (2001) Early-onset amyloid deposition and cognitive deficits in transgenic mice expressing a double mutant form of amyloid precursor protein 695. J Biol Chem 276:21562–21570

Cummings BJ, Pike CJ, Shankle R, Cotman CW (1996) Beta-amyloid deposition and other measures of neuropathology predict cognitive status in Alzheimer's disease. Neurobiol Aging 1:921–933

Haroutunian V, Perl DP, Purohit DP, Marin D, Khan K, Lantz M, Davis KL, Mohs RC (1998) Regional distribution of neuritic plaques in the nondemented elderly and subjects with very mild Alzheimer disease. Arch Neurol 55:1185–1191

Hartley DM, Walsh DM, Ye CP, Diehl T, Vasquez S, Vassilev PM, Teplow DB, Selkoe DJ (1999) Protofibrillar intermediates of amyloid beta-protein induce acute electrophysiological changes and progressive neurotoxicity in cortical neurons. J Neurosci 19:8876–8884

Janus C, Pearson J, McLaurin J, Mathews PM, Jiang Y, Schmidt SD, Chishti MA, Horne P, Heslin D, French J, Mount HTJ, Nixon RA, Mercken M, Bergeron C, Fraser PE, St George-Hyslop P, Westaway D (2000) A beta peptide immunization reduces behavioural impairment and plaques in a model of Alzheimer's disease. Nature 408:979–982

Janus C, Zuker N, Pearson J, Cheung A, Cohen M, McLaurin J, St George-Hyslop P (2001) Water maze search patterns in APP transgenic mice immunised with $A\beta_{42}$ peptide. Soc Neurosci Abstracts 27(Program# 649.5)

Kanne SM, Balota DA, Storandt M, McKeel DWJ, Morris JC (1998) Relating anatomy to function in Alzheimer's disease: neuropsychological profiles predict regional neuropathology 5 years later. Neurology 50:979–985

Katzman TRD, Bick K, Sisodia SS (eds) (1999) Alzheimer Disease (Second ed.) Lippincott, Williams and Wilkins Inc, Baltimore

Lu DC, Rabizadeh S, Chandra S, Shayya RF, Ellerby LM, Ye X, Salvesen GS, Koo EH, Bredesen DE (2000) A second cytotoxic proteolytic peptide derived from amyloid beta-protein precursor. Nature Med 6:397–404

Martin P, Bateson P (1996) Measuring behaviour. Cambridge University Press, Cambridge

McLean CA, Cherny RA, Fraser FW, Fuller SJ, Smith MJ, Beyreuther K, Bush AI, Masters CL (1999) Soluble pool of Abeta amyloid as a determinant of severity of neurodegeneration in Alzheimer's disease. Ann Neurol 46:860–866

Nakagawa Y, Reed L, Nakamura M, McIntosh TK, Smith DH, Saatman KE, Raghupathi R, Clemens J, Saido TC, Lee VM, Trojanowski JQ (2000) Brain trauma in aged transgenic mice induces regression of established abeta deposits. Exp Neurol 163:244–252

Pike CJ, Burdick D, Walencewicz AJ, Glabe CG, Cotman CW (1993) Neurodegeneration induced by beta-amyloid peptides in vitro: the role of peptide assembly state. J Neurosci 13:1676–1687

Schenk D, Barbour R, Dunn W, Gordon G, Grajeda H, Guido T, Hu K, Huang J, Johnson-Wood K, Khan K, Kholodenko D, Lee M, Liao Z, Lieberburg I, Motter R, Mutter L, Soriano F, Shopp G, Vasquez N, Vandevert C, Walker S, Wogulis M, Yednock T, Games D, Seubert P (1999) Immunization with amyloid-beta attenuates Alzheimer-disease-like pathology in the PDAPP mouse. Nature 400:173–177

Steiner H, Capell A, Leimer U, Haass C (1999) Genes and mechanisms involved in beta-amyloid generation and Alzheimer's disease. Eur Arch Psychiatr Clin Neurosci 249:266–270

Walsh DM, Hartley DM, Kusumoto Y, Fezoui Y, Condron MM, Lomakin A, Benedek GB, Selkoe DJ, Teplow DB (1999) Amyloid beta-protein fibrillogenesis. Structure and biological activity of protofibrillar intermediates. J Biol Chem 274:25945–25952

Intranasal Aβ Vaccination as an Approach to Treating β-Amyloidosis

D. J. Selkoe[1]

Summary

The cerebral accumulation of amyloid β-protein (Aβ) in Alzheimer's disease (AD) is accompanied by an inflammatory reaction marked by microgliosis, astrocytosis and the release of pro-inflammatory cytokines and acute phase proteins. Mucosal administration of disease-implicated proteins can induce antigen-specific, anti-inflammatory immune responses in mucosal lymphoid tissue which subsequently act systemically. We hypothesized that chronic mucosal administration of Aβ peptide might induce an anti-inflammatory immune process in which cells induced in the mucosa would circulate to and enter brain tissue to provide a Th2-type cytokine response that could decrease local inflammation. To test this hypothesis, we treated human APP transgenic mice between the ages of ~5 and ~12 months with synthetic human $Aβ_{1-40}$ peptide given mucosally (orally or intranasally) each week. In the mice treated intranasally, we found significant decreases in cerebral Aβ plaque burden as well as $Aβ_{42}$ levels, compared to a control group of mice treated with myelin basic protein or left untreated. The lower Aβ burden in the nasally treated mice was associated with decreased local microglial and astrocytic activation, decreased neuritic dystrophy, serum anti-Aβ antibodies of the IgG1 and IgG2b classes and a small number of mononuclear cells in the brain expressing the anti-inflammatory cytokines, IL-4, IL-10 and TGF-β. Our results demonstrate that chronic nasal administration of Aβ can induce a cellular and humoral immune response to Aβ that decreases cerebral Aβ levels, suggesting a novel mucosal immunological approach for the treatment and prevention of AD.

Introduction

Converging evidence from neuropathological, genetic, cell biology and transgenic modeling studies supports an early, invariant and necessary role for cerebral accumulation of the 42- and 40-residue amyloid β-proteins (Aβ) in the pathogenesis of Alzheimer's disease (AD; Selkoe 2001). The accumulation of $Aβ_{42}$

[1] Center for Neurologic Diseases, Harvard Medical School and Brigham and Women's Hospital, Boston MA 02115, 77 Avenue Louis Pasteur, HIM 730, Phone: 617-525-5200, Fax: 617-525-5252, Email: dselkoe@rics.bwh.harvard.edu

Selkoe/Christen
Immunization Against Alzheimer's Disease
and Other Neurodegenerative Disorders
© Springer-Verlag Berlin Heidelberg 2003

initially in amorphous deposits (diffuse plaques) is followed by the maturation of some of these plaques to forms that include activated microglia, reactive astrocytes (Dickson 1997; Itagaki et al. 1989) and a periplaqueinflammatory response marked by cytokine accumulation [e.g., interleukin (IL-1β, tumor necrosis factor-α; McGeer and McGeer 1995), complement activation (Eikelenboom and Stam 1982; Rogers et al. 1992), and accrual of acute phase proteins (e.g., α1-antichymotrypsin, serum amyloid P component; Abraham et al. 1988; Kalaria et al. 1991). The presence of these changes in AD brain tissue and in relevant transgenic models has led to proposals for anti-inflammatory treatment of the disease, and limited clinical evidence has suggested that this treatment could ultimately prove to be efficacious (Rogers et al. 1993; Stewart et al. 1997).

Chronic mucosal administration of proteins implicated in disease has been shown to decrease organ-specific inflammatory processes in a number of animal models of autoimmune disorders, including those affecting the nervous system (Faria and Weiner 1999). For example, oral or nasal administration of myelin basic protein (MBP; Bitar and Whitacre 1988) or the acetylcholine receptor (Ma et al. 1995; Okumata et al. 1994) has been shown to suppress experimental autoimmune encephalomyelitis and experimental myasthenia gravis, respectively. A principal mechanism by which mucosally administered antigen appears to operateis by inducing anti-inflammatory IL-4/IL-10 [T helper (Th) 2] and tumor growth factor (TGF)-β (Th3) immune responses in mucosal lymphoid tissue, which can then act systemically (Chen et al. 1994). For orally administered proteins, this benefit of mucosal administration is preferentially observed at lower doses (Gregerson et al. 1993; Friedman and Weiner 1994). Based on increasing evidence that local inflammatory processes initiated by Aβ play a modulatory role in AD (McGeer and McGeer 1995; Eikelenboom et al. 1994; Rogers et al. 1996), we conducted experiments to determine whether chronic mucosal administration of Aβ peptide itself could beneficially affect the immunological and neuropathological status of the PDAPP transgenic mouse, an animal model of certain key features of AD (Games et al. 1995; Masliah et al. 1996; Johnson-Wood et al. 1997).

After these experiments were completed, Schenk and coworkers (1999) reported an immunologically based approach for the attenuation of AD-like pathology in the PDAPP mouse model. In their work, repetitive parenteral immunization with Aβ peptide induced a strong humoral immune response that was associated with highly significant decreases in cerebral amyloid deposition and the neuropathological effects thereof. The authors postulated that the beneficial effects they observed were related to the generation of anti-amyloid antibodies which interfered with amyloid deposition and/or enhanced amyloid clearance (Schenk et al. 1999). The results of our study show that chronic nasal administration of Aβ has similar humoral effects and may also involve cellular immune responses. Thus, our findings extend the concept of immunonologically based therapy to the potential treatment of AD through a mucosal route.

Methods and Results

Nasal treatment with Aβ significantly reduces Aβ deposits in brains of PDAPP mice.

In this initial study of our nasal Aβ vaccination approach, we carried out a seven-month mucosal treatment protocol in 52 PDAPP transgenic mice beginning at the age of ~5 months and ending at ~12 months. Doses of synthetic human $Aβ_{1-40}$ peptide were chosen based on pilot experiments in non-transgenic littermates in which oral or nasal Aβ peptide treatment led to a systemic immune response characterized by increases in cells secreting IL-4/IL-10 and TGF-β. The 52 study mice were randomized to three control and four Aβ treatment groups, as follows: group 1, untreated (n = 7); group 2, 500 µg of oral MBP (n = 5); group 3, 50 µg of nasal MBP (n = 6); group 4, 10 µg of oral Aβ peptide (n = 9); group 5, 100 µg of oral Aβ (n = 9); group 6, 5 µg of nasal Aβ (n = 7); and group 7, 25 µg of nasal Aβ (n = 9).

In the first week of treatment, the three oral treatment groups were fed daily with their respective antigens (MBP or human $Aβ_{1-40}$) for five consecutive days, and the three nasal treatment groups were given their respective antigens (MBP or human $Aβ_{1-40}$) intranasally on days 1, 3 and 5. Thereafter, all mice received their respective antigens once per week for a total of ~7 months. Mice were fed Aβ in 0.2 ml of water with a ball-type feeding needle or else underwent nasal instillation of Aβ in 0.01 ml of water.

Following the seven-month treatment protocol (above) and sacrifice at ~12 months of age, all 52 mouse brains underwent extensive immunohistochemical studies, including quantification of Aβ plaque burden by computer-assisted imaging. As has been previously reported (Games et al. 1995; Masliah et al. 1996; Johnson-Wood et al. 1997; Schenk et al. 1999) PDAPP mice showed substantial individual variation (up to nine-fold) in the amounts of Aβ deposits developing during the course of their cerebral β-amyloidosis. Therefore, some mice in each of our seven treatment groups had low, medium or high numbers of Aβ deposits in hippocampus and adjacent cerebral cortex (Fig. 1). Computerized image analysis performed simultaneously on Aβ-immunostained brain sections of all 52 mice established the precise amounts of Aβ deposits in the hippocampus. The three control groups showed no significant differences in the mean percentages of Aβ burden: 3.31 ± 2.35% in the seven untreated mice; 5.78 ± 2.97% in the five mice in the oral MBP-treated group; and 3.87 ± 4.86% in the six mice in the nasal MBP-treated group. In view of the lack of effect of MBP treatment, the large Aβ variation among individual mice (Fig. 1) and the limited number of mice available to us for study, we compared each of the four Aβ peptide treatment groups with the mice in these three combined control groups, using a conservative statistical method, the two-tailed Mann-Whitney U test (J. Orav, Department of Biostatistics, Brigham and Women's Hospital). Computer-assisted image analysis revealed that the mice treated intranasally with Aβ peptide at a dose of 25 µg/wk (group 7) had a substantial (~60%) and statistically significant ($p<0.037$) decrease in mean hippocampal Aβ plaque burden: 1.72 ± 1.39% (n = 9), compared with that of the controls: 4.18 ± 3.47% (n =18; Table 1 and Fig. 2).

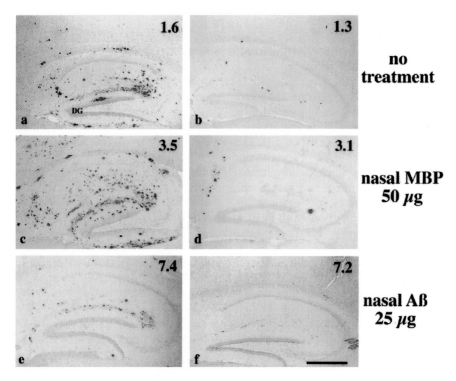

Fig. 1. Variability of Aβ plaque burden in PDAPP transgenic mice at age 12 months. Immuno-histochemistry with an antiserum to human Aβ (R1282) on hippocampal sections of representative mice from treatment groups 1 (untreated), 3 (nasal MBP 50 μg) and 7 (nasal Aβ 25 μg). Left panels show the mice with the highest Aβ burdens within each of these three groups; right panels show the mice with the lowest Aβ burdens (numbers refer to individual mice). The lower Aβ burden documented in group 7 mice (Table 1) can be seen by comparing these three highest and three lowest animals. DG, dentate gyrus. Hematoxylin counterstained. Bar, 500 μm.

The mice in the 5 μg/wk nasal Aβ peptide group also showed a lower mean Aβ-immunoreactive area in hippocampus (2.27 ± 2.41%; n = 7) than did the controls (4.18 ± 3.47%; n =18), but the difference did not reach statistical significance (Table 1 and Fig. 2). However, a comparison between all the mice treated nasally with Aβ peptide (n =16) and all the control mice (n =18) showed a significant decrease (p<0.037) in mean hippocampal Aβ plaque burden in the former. Comparison between the two Aβ orally treated groups (either individually or combined) and the 18 control mice showed no statistically significant decrease or increase in mean Aβ plaque burden as a result of oral exposure. When we quantified Aβ burden a second time by computer-assisted imaging in a combined area of hippocampus and adjacent temporal cortex in new brain sections, we again observed a significant decrease in mean Aβ burden selectively in the nasal 25 μg/wk nasal Aβ group compared to the controls (p<0.04, one-tailed Mann-Whitney U test).

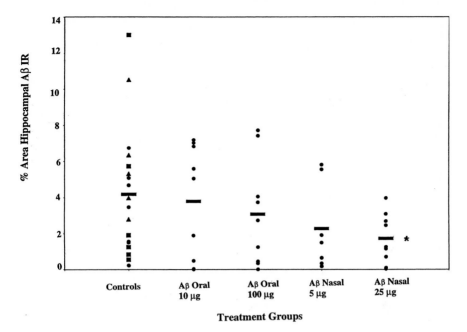

Fig 2. Scatter plot of hippocampal Aβ plaque burden for all 52 mice as measured by computer assisted imaging (see Methods). Controls include untreated mice (circles) and mice treated with either oral MBP 500 μg (squares) or nasal MBP 50 μg (triangles). * Mean for Aβ nasal 25 μg mice differs significantly from the controls (p<0.037).

Table 1. Nasal and oral treatment with Aβ

Group	Aβ plaque burden in hippocampus[a]	Aβ X-42 levels in brain[b]	Presence of anti-Aβ Cellular immune	
			antibodies	changes in brain
Control	4.18 ± 3.47 (n=18)	592 ± 383 (n=8)	0/16	None[c]
Oral Aβ (10 μg)	3.79 ± 3.14 (n=9)	763 ± 566 (n=4)	2/9	None
Oral Aβ (100 μg)	3.08 ± 2.95 (n=9)	661 ± 477 (n=4)	1/9	None
Nasal Aβ (5 μg)	2.27 ± 2.41 (n=7)	396 ± 280 (n=3)	4/7	None
Nasal Aβ (25 μg)	1.72 ± 1.39 (n=9)[d]	282 ± 187 (n=4)[e]	8/9[f]	Mononuclear cell infiltration with cytokine expression (IL-4, IL-10, TGFβ)

[a] Percentage Aβ immune reactivity; mean ± SD
[b] pmol/g; mean ± SD
[c] Rare mononuclear cells, no cytokine expression
[d] p < 0.037 vs. control (2-tailed Mann-Whitney U test)
[e] p < 0.033 vs. control (repeated measures ANOVA)
[f] p < 0.0001 vs. control (Fisher's exact test 2-tailed)
Aβ = amyloid β-peptide; IL – interleukin; TGF = tumor growth factor

Quantification of Cerebral Aβ_{42} by ELISA Confirms the Aβ-Lowering Effect of Chronic Nasal Aβ Treatment

Sensitive sandwich ELISAs for Aβ (Johnson-Wood et al. 1997; Seubert et al. 1992) were carried out on the entire contralateral (frozen) hemisphere of representative mouse brains from each of the seven treatment groups. This method measures the total Aβ content of the brain tissue, whereas the anti-Aβ image analysis measures just that Aβ deposited within microscopically recognizable plaques. It should be noted that brain levels of APP were the same in all treatment groups, as expected. We measured Aβ species referred to as X-42 and X-40, which are peptides that begin anywhere in the N-terminal region of Aβ and end at either the 42nd or 40th residue, respectively.

The mean levels of Aβ_{X-42} among the three control groups of mice (untreated: 453 $\pm$ 96 pmol/g; oral MBP: 887 $\pm$ 584 pmol/g; nasal MBP: 535 $\pm$ 460 pmol/g) showed no statistical difference from each other. The brains of the 25 µg/wk Aβ nasally treated mice measured by ELISA (n = 4) contained a mean of 282 $\pm$ 187 pmol/g of Aβ_{X-42}, representing a 52% decrease (p<0.033; repeated-measures ANOVA) compared to the mean of 592 $\pm$ 383 pmol/g for the control mice (n = 8; (Table 1). When we compared mean Aβ_{X-42} level of the 25 µg/wk Aβ nasal mice (282 $\pm$ 187 pmol/g) solely to that of the mice who had received no treatment (453 $\pm$ 96 pmol/g), a significant 38% decrease (p < 0.044) was observed. The mean Aβ_{X-42} level of the 5 µg Aβ nasal mice was 396 $\pm$ 280 pmol/g, a 33% decrease from the mean level of the controls that did not reach statistical significance.

As in the case of Aβ computer-assisted imaging (previous section), Aβ_{X-42} ELISA showed no significant changes in brain Aβ levels in either of the oral Aβ treated groups (10 µg/wk oral Aβ: 763 $\pm$ 566 pmol/g; 100 µg/wk oral Aβ: 661 $\pm$ 477 pmol/g), compared with controls (592 $\pm$ 383 pmol/g). Although the far less abundant Aβ_{X-40} species in the mouse brain was somewhat decreased in the 25 µg/wk nasal Aβ (16 $\pm$ 10 pmol/g) versus control mice (24 $\pm$ 12 pmol/g), the difference was not significant. The mean Aβ amounts determined by ELISA in each of the seven treatment groups correlated well with the mean amounts of deposited Aβ as determined by computerized image analysis. Furthermore, our ELISA values in the control mice are in the same range as those reported previously in untreated PDAPP mice of this age (Johnson-Wood et al. 1997)

Decreased Aβ Deposition in Nasally Treated Mice is Associated With Decreased Microgliosis, Astrocytosis and Neuritic Dystrophy

Our initial hypothesis was that chronic mucosal Aβ administration might decrease the inflammatory cytopathology that occurs in and around Aβ plaques. To address this question, we stained sections of all 52 brains with antibodies to the microglial surface antigens, CD45 (leukocyte common antigen) and CD11b (Mac-1). We also probed with anti-GFAP antiserum. In all seventreatment groups, the pattern of activated microglia closely paralleled that of Aβ plaques: mice with few Aβ deposits in hippocampus and adjacent cerebral cortex showed correspondingly low numbers of active microglia in these areas, and vice versa. This finding

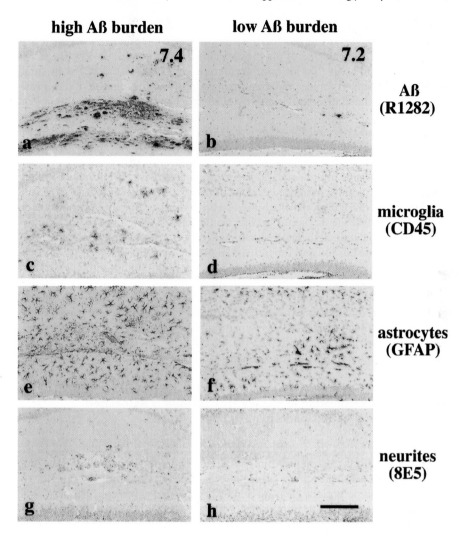

Fig. 3. Immunohistochemistry demonstrates correlation between Aβ deposition and various markers of plaque-associated inflammation in hippocampi of PDAPP mice chronically treated with nasal Aβ 25 µg (group 7). **a, c, e** and **g**: serial sections from mouse 7.4, with the highest Aβ plaque burden in group 7. **b, d, f** and **h**: serial sections from mouse 7.2, with the lowest Aβ plaque burden in group 7. **a, b**: Aβ (R1282). **c, d**: microglia (CD45). **e, f**: astrocytes (GFAP). **g, h**: APP-immunoreactive dystrophic neurites (8E5). Bar, 200 µm.

was illustrated in the nine mice in the 25 µg/wk nasal Aβ treatment group. Those animals with substantial numbers of hippocampal and neocortical Aβ deposits also retained numerous plaque-associated activated microglia, whereas most of the mice in this Aβ nasal group, which had low Aβ burdens (Fig. 2), also had little microgliosis (Fig. 3a–d). Plaque-associated reactive astrocytes in hippocampus were far fewer in mice with low numbers of Aβ deposits, regardless of treatment group, and vice versa (Fig. 3e,f). The same correlation applied in the neocortex. Complement C1q, a marker of plaque-associated inflammation in AD (Rogers et al. 1992) as well as in PDAPP mice (Lemere et al. 1998), was detected in small numbers of plaques in mice of all treatment groups, and the amount of C1q staining again correlated directly with Aβ plaque burden, regardless of treatment (not shown).

Next, we asked whether the apparent clearing of Aβ deposits and the resultant decrease in local microglial and astrocytic reactions were associated with any adverse neuropathological consequences in the regions now largely lacking plaques. Sections of hippocampus and adjacent neocortex were immunolabeled for synaptophysin, a phosphorylated epitope of neuronal tau protein (Mab AT8), and for APP (Mab 8E5), both of which are sensitive markers for injured neurites in AD as well as transgenic mouse brains (Games et al. 1995). As in the case of the glial markers, plaque-associated neuritic alteration again corresponded directly to the Aβ plaque burden and the individual plaque morphology, regardless of experimental treatment group (Fig. 3g, h). Those mice with high Aβ plaque burdens had more neuritic plaques, with the staining of dystrophic neurites by antibodies AT8 and 8E5 occurring mostly in areas of compacted plaques. We observed no increase in abnormal neurites in Aβ nasally treated animals with low plaque numbers. Indeed, these mice had less synaptophysin-, tau- and APP-positive dystrophic neurites than mice with high plaque burdens (Fig. 3g, h), in keeping with the decreased glial responses in the former.

Decreased Aβ Deposition in Nasally Treated Mice is Associated with Circulating Aβ Antibodies

We analyzed whether the significant decrease in brain Aβ levels observed in the 25 µg/wk nasal Aβ treatment group was associated with a humoral response to the peptide. To ascertain the presence of bona fide Aβ antibodies capable of reacting with and potentially clearing brain Aβ deposits, we screened the sera of all 52 mice for their ability to immunolabel typical Aβ plaques in the brains of humans with AD or Down's syndrome/AD (Fig. 4; see Table 1). Almost all (eight of nine) mice in the 25 µg/wk nasal Aβ group had readily detectable titers of antibodies to human Aβ, ranging between 1:1000 and 1:50,000 (as determined by serial dilution and immunoreaction on AD brain sections;Table 1 and Fig. 4a, c and e). Several mice (four of seven) in the 5 µg/wk nasal Aβ treatment group also showed plaque immunolabeling by their sera (Table 1 and Fig. 4d). Only one of the 100 µg/wk oral Aβ mice and two of the 10 µg/wk oral Aβ mice had anti-Aβ antibodies in their sera (Table 1 and Fig. 4b), and these were present at low titers. No Aβ antibodies were detected in mice that had not been treated with Aβ.

We next established a sensitive ELISA for measuring anti-Aβ antibodies in the mouse sera. This analysis provided levels ranging between 0.1 and 54.6 µg/ml in the eight immunopositive mice of group 7 (Aβ 25 µg/wk treatment group). In six of the nine 25 µg/wk nasal Aβ treated mice, the Aβ antibody level determined by ELISA showed a rough inverse correlation with the hippocampal plaque burden,

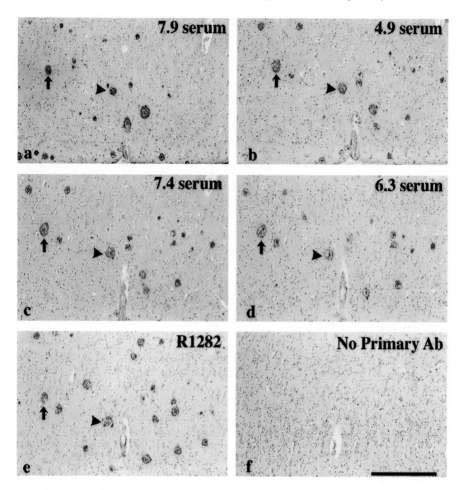

Fig. 4. Chronic nasal treatment of PDAPP mice with Aβ induces anti-Aβ antibodies. **a-d:** Sera from the four mice indicated were diluted at 1:100 and used as primary antibodies to immunolabel amyloid plaques in serial brain sections from a 92-year-old patient with typical AD. **e:** Reference Aβ antiserum R1282 produces identical staining. Arrows and arrowheads indicate a few of the many plaques labeled by all the antisera. **f:** No primary antibody control. Bar **a-f:** 400 μm.

as determined by computer-assisted imaging, whereas in the other three mice, no clear correlation was apparent. The Aβ antibodies were predominantly of the IgG1 and IgG2b class, both of which are characteristic of Th2 type immune responses. Preabsorption of each immunopositive mouse serum with synthetic Aβ peptide abolished the staining. It should be noted that the anti-Aβ antibodies in the immunopositive mouse sera did not react with full-length human or mouse APP on Western blots or with mouse synthetic Aβ peptide, as expected for most antibodies raised against human $A\beta_{1-40}$.

Decreased Aβ Deposition in Nasally Treated Mice is Associated with Mononuclear Cells Expressing IL-4, IL-10 and TGF-β in the Brain

We asked whether mucosal treatment with Aβ peptide resulted in cellular immune activity in the brain. The presence or absence of mononuclear cell infiltration was assessed in a blinded fashion; immunohistochemistry for cells expressing IFN-γ, IL-2, IL-4, IL-10, and TGF-β was performed in one half of the mice in each treatment group. No immunoreactive mononuclear cells were observed in the untreated (group 1) or in MBP-treated (groups 2 and 3) or oral Aβ treated (groups 4 and 5) mice. In four of the five mice examined for mononuclear cells in the 25 μg/wk nasal Aβ treatment group, a very small number of mononuclear cells that included cells immunoreactive for IL-4, IL-10 and TGF-β antibodies were observed within and surrounding the hippocampus (data not shown). Analysis of serially stained sections demonstrated that most such cells were T cells and included both CD4 and CD8 cells (not shown). While these mononuclear cells were observed in plaque-containing regions of the brain, they showed no specific relationship to the plaques themselves. We detected no cells expressing IL-2 or IFN-γ.

Discussion

In this work, we demonstrate the novel finding that chronic nasal administration of human Aβ$_{1-40}$ peptide to mice transgenic for human APP results in a significant, roughly 50% decrease in Aβ accumulation and deposition in the brain and a resultant decrease in plaque-associated microgliosis, astrocytosis and neuritic dystrophy. This effect was specifically associated with an anti-Aβ antibody response and with a modest mononuclear cell infiltration in the brain.

We initially hypothesized that repetitive mucosal administration of Aβ might lead to anti-inflammatory Th2-type immune responses that could decrease the local inflammation and plaque maturation occurring in the PDAPP mouse model. In testing this hypothesis, we found that weekly nasal administration of Aβ peptide for seven months lowered Aβ burden in the brains of these mice, which have amyloid pathology similar to that of AD. Rather than finding a stable level of Aβ plaques and a specific decrease in peri-plaque inflammatory markers, we saw an overall decrease in Aβ plaque burden (as measured by image analysis and ELISA), with residual plaques still associated with peri-plaque microgliosis and astrocytosis as well as some neuritic dystrophy. The Aβ-lowering effect of nasal Aβ immunization was strongly associated with an Aβ antibody response. These results are thus consistent with and extend those of Schenk et al. (1999). Thus, we conclude that Aβ nasal immunization has beneficial effects, but apparently by raising an anti-Aβ immunological response that includes a prominent humoral component, rather than by suppressing inflammation around existing plaques.

Although the number of PDAPP mice available for this study was small, it is important to note that both the humoral and cellular immunological responses were observed specifically in the one treatment group that showed significant reductions in cerebral Aβ, as measured by quantitative imaging and ELISA (see Table 1). In other words, a significant decrease in mean Aβ burden occurred selectively in that treatment group that developed anti-human Aβ antibodies and a limited cellular anti-inflammatory cytokine response in the brain. In this initial study, chronic oral administration of Aβ produced very few or no anti-Aβ antibodies or a detectable cellular immune response in the brain. Accordingly, this lack of immune response to chronic oral Aβ administration was associated with a lack of decrease in mean cerebral Aβ, as detected by both image analysis and ELISA. Oral or nasal administration of another brain protein, MBP, had no effect. Therefore, it is very likely that the humoral and cellular responses observed selectively in the Aβ nasally treated animals are causally related to the significantly lower brain Aβ levels seen only in these mice.

The secretion of IL-4, IL-10 and TGF-β by a small number of mononuclear cells induced by nasal Aβ peptide treatment and present in the brain could interfere with Aβ aggregation or stabilization in brain tissue and/or enhance its clearance. In this regard, the local brain inflammatory responses believed to be triggered by Aβ may contribute to further Aβ aggregation and the formation of stable deposits (McGeer and McGeer 1995; Rogers et al. 1996).

Our results using nasal Aβ treatment in these mice need to be interpreted in light of the fact that cerebral Aβ burden varies greatly among individual PDAPP mice. For example, control (PBS-injected) PDAPP mice in the study of Schenk and coworkers were found to show as much as a nine-fold variation in the amount of Aβ immunoreactive area in the brain (Schenk et al. 1999). We observed this same large variation in both our control and treatment groups. Despite the large variance, the mean Aβ burden in our 25 μg/wk nasal Aβ treatment group was significantly decreased from that in the control animals.

An interpretation of our own results consistent with that of Schenk and coworkers (1999) is that the occurrence of anti-Aβ antibodies in our chronic nasal Aβ-treated animals is the basis for the substantial (50–60%) reduction in mean cerebral Aβ levels seen selectively in this treatment group. The titer of anti-Aβ antibodies achieved by repetitive parenteral immunizations is far higher than that which occurs by the mucosal route. Nonetheless, the relatively modest Aβ titers in the sera of our mice were apparently sufficient to produce substantial and statistically significant clearing of Aβ deposits.

Future mouse experiments investigating mucosal therapy given several times per week and beginning at earlier ages are likely to yield stronger biological effects. In this regard, the work of Lemere and colleagues (in this volume) substantially extends the nasal Aβ treatment approach first described in this study. Our results also raise the possibility that the generation of immune cells specific for Aβ could play a role in the Aβ-lowering response. It has been reported that cells specific for brain antigens can affect CNS pathological features (Moalem et al. 1999). In the work of Schenk et al. (1999) only antibodies were measured, but the immunization protocol they employed would have led to the generation of a cell-mediated immune response against Aβ as well.

In conclusion, it appears that chronic nasal administration of Aβ is accompanied by the induction of Th2-type antibody responses and Th2-type cellular responses that are associated with a substantial and significant reduction in Aβ burden in the brain. The induction of immune responses by mucosal administration of a synthetic peptide is a relatively safe treatment that can be administered for long periods of time (Faria and Weiner 1999), making it applicable to a chronic disease such as AD. The beneficial results obtained in this study occurred in the absence of any adjuvant administration. Nonetheless, the use of adjuvants has recently been shown to substantially potentiate the effect of intranasal Aβ (see Lemere et al., this volume). Furthermore, the principally Th2-type responses generated by chronic mucosal administration of an antigen might be potentially less likely to induce harmful side effects that Th1-type immune response would. The treatment or prevention of AD using a mucosal route for Aβ administration might be better tolerated in human patients than repetitive parenteral administration in the presence of adjuvant. It is also possible that an initial parenteral immunization followed by chronic intranasal administration would prove useful. The central issue that remains unanswered here is the degree to which results in this mouse model are relevant to treatment of AD in humans. Only clinical trials of nasal Aβ can answer this question.

[Note: This chapter is adapted from in Weiner et al, Ann. Neurol, 48:567–579, 2000]

References

Abraham CR, Selkoe DJ, Potter H (1988) Immunochemical identification of the serine protease inhibitor, α1-antichymotrypsin in the brain amyloid deposits of Alzheimer's disease. Cell 52:487–501

Bitar DM, Whitacre CC (1988) Suppression of experimental autoimmune encephalomyelitis by the oral administration of myelin basic protein. Cell Immunol 112:364–370

Chen Y, Kuchroo VK, Inobe J-I, Hafler DA, Weiner HL (1994) Regulatory T-cell clones induced by oral tolerance: suppression of autoimmune encephalomyelitis. Science 265:1237–1240

Dickson DW (1997) The pathogenesis of senile plaques. J Neuropathol Exp Neurol 56:321–339

Eikelenboom P, Stam FC (1982) Immunoglobulins and complement factors in senile plaques: an immunoperoxidase study. Acta Neuropathol 57:239–242

Eikelenboom P, Zhan SS, van Gool WA, Allstop D (1994) Inflammatory mechanisms in Alzheimer's disease. Trends Pharmacol Sci 15:447–450

Faria AMC, Weiner HL (1999) Oral tolerance: mechanisms and therapeutic applications. Adv Immunol 73:153–264

Friedman A, Weiner H (1994) Induction of anergy or active suppression following oral tolerance is determined by antigen dosage. Proc Natl Acad Sci USA 91:6688–6692

Games D, Adams D, Alessandrini R, Barbour R, Berthelette P, Blackwell C, Carr T, Clemens J, Donaldson T, Gillespie F, Guido T, Hagopian S, Johnson-Wood K, Khan K, Lee M, Leibowitz P, Lieberburg I, Little S, Masliah E, McConlogue L, Montoya-Zavala M, Mucke L, Paganini L, Penniman E, Power M, schenk D, Seubert P, Snyder B, Soriano F, Tan H, Vitale J, Wadsworth S, Wolozin B, Zhao J (1995) Alzheimer-type neuropathology in transgenic mice overexpressing V717F β-amyloid precursor protein. Nature 373:523–527

Gregerson DS, Obritsch WF, Donoso LA (1993) Oral tolerance in experimental autoimmune uveoretinitis. Distinct mechanisms of resistance are induced by low dose vs high dose feeding protocols. J Immunol 151:5751–5761

Higgins P, Weiner HL (1988) Suppression of experimental autoimmune encephalomyelitis by oral administration of myelin basic protein and its fragments. J Immunol 140:440–445

Itagaki S, McGeer PL, Akiyama H, Zhu S, Selkoe D (1989) Relationship of microglia and astro-cytes to amyloid deposits of Alzheimer disease. J Neuroimmunol 24:173–182

Johnson-Wood K, Lee M, Motter R, Hu K, Gordon G, Barbour R, Khan K, Gordon M, Tan H, Games D, Lieberburg I, Schenk D, Seubert P, McConlogue L (1997) Amyloid precursor pro-tein processing and Aβ42 deposition in a transgenic mouse model of Alzheimer disease. Proc Natl Acad Sci USA 94:1550–1555

Kalaria RN, Galloway PG, Perry G (1991) Widespread amyloid P component immunoreactivity in cortical amyloid deposits of Alzheimer's disease and other degenerative disorders. Neu-ropathol Appl Neurobiol 17:189–201

Lemere C, Grenfell T, Mori C, Stoltzner S, Khan K, Bales K, Games D, Selkoe DJ (1998) Temporal accrual of inflammatory proteins in the plaques of PD-APP transgenic mice between 8 and 20 months. Neurobiol. Aging 19:S279

Ma C-G, Zhang G-X, Xiao B-G, Olsson T, Link H (1995) Suppression of experimental autoim-mune myasthenia gravis by nasal administration of acetylcholine receptor. J Neuroimmunol 58:51–60

Masliah E, Sisk A, Mallory M, Mucke L, Schenk D, Games D (1996) Comparison of neurodegen-erative pathology in transgenic mice overexpressing V717F β-amyloid precursor protein and Alzheimer's disease. J. Neurosci. 16:5795–5811

McGeer PL, McGeer EG (1995) The inflammatory response system of brain: implications for therapy of Alzheimer and other neurodegenerative diseases. Brain Res Rev 21:195–218

Metzler B, Wraith DC (1993) Inhibition of experimental autoimmune encephalomyelitis by inhalation but not oral administration of the encephalitogenic peptide: influence of MHC binding affinity. Int Immunol 5:1159–1165

Moalem G, Leibowitz-Amit R, Yoles E, Mor F, Cohen IR, Schwartz M (1999) Autoimmune T cells protect neurons from secondary degeneration after central nervous system axotomy. Nature Med 5:49–55

Okumura S, McIntosh K, Drachman DB (1994) Oral administration of acetylcholine receptor: effects on experimental myasthenia gravis. Ann Neurol 36:704–713

Rogers J, Cooper NR, Webster S, J Schultz, PL McGeer, SD Styren, WH Civin, L Brachova, B Bradt, P Ward , I Lieberburg (1992) Complement activation by β-amyloid in Alzheimer disease. Proc Natl Acad Sci USA 89:10016–10020

Rogers J, Kirby LC, Hempelman SR, Berry DL, McGeer PL, Kaszniak AW, Zalinski J, Cofield M, Mansukhani L, Willson P (1993) Clinical trial of indomethacin in Alzheimer's disease. Neu-rology 43:1609–1611

Rogers J, Webster S, Lue L-F, Brachova L, Civin WH, Emmerling M, Shivers B, Walker D, McGeer P (1996) Inflammation and Alzheimer's disease pathogenesis. Neurobiol Aging 17:681–686

Schenk D, Barbour R, Dunn W, Gordon G, Grajeda H, Guido T, Hu K, Huang J, Johnson-Wood K, Khan K, Kholodenko D, Lee M, Liao Z, Lieberburg I, Motter R, Mutter L, Soriano F, Shopp G, Vasquez N, Vandevert C, Walker S, Wogulis M, Yednock T, Games D, Seubert P (1999) Immu-nization with amyloid-β attenuates Alzheimer-disease-like pathology in the PDAPP mouse. Nature 400:173–177

Selkoe DJ (2001) Alzheimer's disease: genes, proteins and therapies. Physiol Rev 81:742–761

Seubert P, Vigo-Pelfrey C, Esch F, Lee M, Dovey H, Davis D, Sinha S, Schlossmacher M, Whaley J, Swindlehurst C, McCormack R, Wolfert R, Selkoe D, Lieberburg I, Schenk D 1992) Isolation and quantitation of soluble Alzheimer's β-peptide from biological fluids. Nature 359:325–327

Stewart WF, Kawas C, Corrada M, Metter EJ (1997) Risk of Alzheimer's disease and duration of NSAID use. Neurology 48:626–632

Weiner HL, Lemere CA, Maron R, Spooner ET, Grenfell TJ, Mori C, Issazadeh S, Hancock WW, Selkoe DJ (2000) Nasal administration of amyloid-β peptide decreases cerebral amyloid bur-den in a mouse model of Alzheimer's disease. Ann Neurol 48:567–579

Improvements in Intranasal Amyloid-β (Aβ) Immunization in Mice

C. A. Lemere[1], E. T. Spooner[1], J. F. Leverone[1], J. D. Clements[2]*

Summary

Previously, we showed that intranasal (i.n.) administration of Aβ1-40 in PDAPP mice for seven months led to a 58% decrease in cerebral Aβ burden (Weiner et al. 2000; Lemere et al. 2000). Serum anti-Aβ titers were low. Since then, we have focused on optimizing our i.n. Aβ immunization protocol using different routes of administration – a proven mucosal adjuvant, *Escherichia coli* heat-labile enterotoxin (LT), and various Aβ peptides as immunogens – in an effort to increase Aβ antibody titers. First, we compared three routes of Aβ immunization [intraperitoneal (i.p.) injection, i.n. administration and a combination thereof] in two strains of wild type (WT) mice. B6D2F1 mice were much more responsive to Aβ immunization than were C56BL/6 mice; i.p. Aβ immunization and the combination of i.p. with i.n. Aβ gave the highest titers. Second, when low doses of the mucosal adjuvant LT were given with Aβ i.n., there was a dramatic, 12-fold increase in Aβ antibody titers in B6D2F1 mice treated two times a week for eight weeks compared to those of mice receiving i.n. Aβ without adjuvant. A non-toxic, mutant form of LT, designated LT(R192G), showed even better adjuvanticity; anti-Aβ antibody titers were 16-fold higher than those seen in mice given i.n. Aβ without adjuvant. Third, in another study, B6D2F1 mice were given i.n. Aβ1-40/42 or Aβ1-15, each with LT(R192G) twice a week for six weeks. Mice receiving full-length Aβ + LT(R192G) generated serum anti-Aβ antibodies earlier and in much greater abundance than did mice given Aβ1-15 + LT(R192G). Mouse serum anti-Aβ antibodies consistently detected human Alzheimer's disease (AD) plaques, had an epitope(s) within Aβ1-15, and were of IgG1 and IgG2b isotypes without adjuvant, but included IgG2a and low levels of IgA with adjuvant. Both forms of LT were well tolerated by the mice and showed no obvious toxic effects. Human Aβ peptide was not detected in any of the mouse brains. More recently, we immunized five PSAPP transgenic (tg) mice, an accelerated mouse model of AD, by giving a

[1] Center for Neurologic Diseases, Brigham & Women's Hospital, Harvard Medical School, Boston, MA 02115

[2] Department of Microbiology and Immunology, Program in Molecular Pathogenesis and Immunity, Tulane University School of Medicine, New Orleans, LA 70112.

[*] Please send correspondence to: Cynthia A. Lemere, Ph.D., Center for Neurologic Diseases, Harvard Institutes of Medicine, Room 622, 77 Avenue Louis Pasteur, Boston, MA 02115, Phone: (617) 525-5214, FAX: (617) 525-5252, E-mail: lemere@cnd.bwh.harvard.edu

Selkoe/Christen
Immunization Against Alzheimer's Disease
and Other Neurodegenerative Disorders
© Springer-Verlag Berlin Heidelberg 2003

single i.p. injection of Aβ1-40/42 + Complete Freund Adjuvant (CFA) at the beginning of the study, followed by i.n. Aβ1-40/42 + LT twice weekly for eight weeks. Immunization was started at five weeks of age, prior to plaque formation. Serum anti-Aβ antibody titers were ~ nine-fold higher than those generated in our earlier study in PDAPP mice. As in the studies above in WT mice, the anti-Aβ antibodies had epitope(s) within Aβ1-15 and were of Ig isotypes IgG2b, IgG2 a and IgG1 in Aβ immunized mice. Serum anti-Aβ titers were not detected in control PSAPP mice. Aβ immunized mice showed significant decreases in cerebral Aβ levels; a 75% decrease in plaque number and a 58% decrease in brain Aβx-42 by ELISA were observed. Gliosis and neuritic dystrophy were limited to the remaining, limited number of plaques. Vehicle controls showed no abnormal brain pathology, indicating the lack of overt inflammation due to treatment with LT. Morphological changes were absent from kidney, spleen and snout. A 28-fold increase in serum Aβ (total) protein levels was observed in Aβ immunized PSAPP mice compared to serum Aβ in control PSAPP mice; most of the Aβ in serum of Aβ immunized mice was complexed to antibodies. We conclude that prime/boost Aβ protocols with adjuvant lead to increased Aβ antibody titers and that the anti-Aβ antibodies may stabilize Aβ in the serum or clear it from the brain.

Introduction

Alzheimer's disease (AD) is the most common form of neurodegenerative disease in the world, and yet there is no effective treatment or cure. Therapeutic strategies aimed at lowering cerebral amyloid-β protein (Aβ) have become increasingly important in AD research for several reasons: 1) Aβ deposition into plaques is one of the earliest pathological changes in AD and represents one of the hallmark lesions of the disease; 2) Aβ neurotoxicity has been demonstrated in vitro and in vivo; and 3) human familial mutations in the amyloid precursor protein (APP) gene and the presenilin (PS1, PS2) genes lead to increased Aβ levels (Selkoe 1999). Examples of these AD prevention and treatment strategies include Aβ vaccination, inhibition of Aβ-generating secretases, and the use of cholesterol-lowering drugs and copper/zinc chelators. Our work focuses on Aβ vaccination.

In 1999, Schenk and colleagues were the first to report the benefits of Aβ vaccination. They showed that chronic Aβ i.p. injections with CFA almost completely prevented plaque deposition in PDAPP mice, a mouse model of AD, when given prior to plaque formation, and dramatically lowered brain Aβ levels if given after plaque deposition had begun (Schenk et al. 1999). Chronic passive transfer of particular Aβ antibodies in PDAPP mice also decreased cerebral Aβ levels (Bard et al. 2000); these authors provided data suggestive of a mechanism wherein Aβ antibodies cross the blood-brain-barrier, bind the Fc-receptor on microglial cells and induce phagocytosis of Aβ.

A number of research groups have since confirmed that Aβ immunization results in a significant reduction in cerebral Aβ levels in APP and PSAPP tg mice and, in some studies, have shown improvement in cognitive deficits. We reported a 56% decrease in cerebral Aβ levels in PDAPP mice and low Aβ antibody titers following weekly i.n. administration of Aβ1-40 between 5 and 12 months of age (Weiner et al. 2000; Lemere et al. 2000). These antibodies recognized an epitope in the amino-terminus of Aβ and were of immunoglobulin (Ig) isotypes IgG1 and IgG2b. Two studies reported protection from cognitive deficits following Aβ immunization in several different AD mouse models (Janus et al. 2000; Morgan et al. 2000). In another study, local application of specific Aβ antibodies to the brain surface led to significant clearance of Aβ plaques, as assessed by multiphoton imaging in the brains of live PDAPP mice (Bacskai et al. 2001). Newer formulations of Aβ as an immunogen include genetically engineered filamentous phages displaying the Aβ3-6 epitope (EFRH; Frenkel et al. 2000), a soluble non-aggregating/non-toxic form of Aβ (Sigurdsson et al. 2001), and microparticle-encapsulated Aβ (Brayden et al. 2001). In 2001, DeMattos and Holtzman suggested another potential mechanism for the cerebral Aβ-clearing effects of Aβ immunization. Their group demonstrated a substantial increase in plasma Aβ following acute, passive transfer of an Aβ monoclonal antibody in PDAPP mice, indicating that the antibodies acted as a "peripheral sink" to clear Aβ from the CNS to the blood (DeMattos et al. 2001).

The following is a review of our more recent studies in which we sought to optimize our Aβ i.n. immunization protocol in WT mice and then apply the new and improved protocol to a study of Aβ immunization in PSAPP double transgenic mice (Holcomb et al. 1998), an AD mouse model with accelerated amyloid pathogenesis. For each of these studies, a cocktail of Aβ peptides [3 parts Aβ1-40 and one part Aβ1-42; Biopolymer Laboratories, Center for Neurologic Diseases (CND), Boston, MA] was diluted at 4 mg/ml in distilled water and incubated overnight at $37°$ C prior to being used as the immunogen. Congo red staining showed minimal fibrils. A shorter peptide, Aβ1-15, was also synthesized by the Biopolymer lab and did not form fibrils. Because many of the AD tg mouse models are generated from mice of various genetic backgrounds, we asked if different strains of mice would respond differently to Aβ immunization. Mouse strain differences have been reported to lead to variability in immune responses to antigens, such as to OVA (Morokata et al. 1999). In addition, we compared routes of Aβ immunization (i.p. vs. i.n. vs. a combination). Next, we asked if the proven mucosal adjuvants LT or a non-toxic mutant form, LT(R192G), would be effective in increasing Aβ antibody titers when given intranasally with Aβ peptide. Based on the knowledge that the Aβ antibodies generated by Aβ immunization recognized an epitope in the amino-terminus of Aβ, we compared full-length Aβ and a shorter fragment (Aβ1-15) as immunogens. Lastly, we immunized PSAPP mice with a single i.p. injection of Aβ with CFA and then chronically boosted the mice with i.n. Aβ with LT twice weekly for eight weeks. Aβ antibody titers were measured in serum; Aβ protein levels were measured in brain and serum.

Optimization of Aβ Immunization Protocols

Differences in Mouse Strain and Protocols

Aβ antibody titers were relatively low in our first study of i.n. Aβ immunization in PDAPP mice; therefore, we compared the timing of Aβ antibody production and titer levels, as well as epitope(s) and Ig isotypes, by immunizing two strains of WT mice (C57BL/6 and B6D2F1) using each of five treatment protocols: 1) chronic i.n. Aβ (without adjuvant); 2) chronic i.p. injections of Aβ (+ CFA/IFA); 3) a single i.p. injection of CFA (without Aβ) to induce an immune response followed by chronic i.n. Aβ; 4. concurrent i.n. Aβ and i.p. Aβ (+ CFA/IFA); and, 5) untreated controls (Spooner et al., 2002). Nasal treatments involved three treatments of 100 μg of Aβ1-40/42 weekly; i.p. injections of 100 μg of Aβ1-40/42 + 50 μg CFA/IFA were given once – per-week. B6D2F1 mice generated Aβ antibodies earlier (after two to three weeks) and in higher quantities than the C57BL/6 mice, indicating that the former were more responsive to Aβ immunization. At the end of the study, ELISA data revealed higher Aβ titers for B6D2F1 mice compared to those of C57BL/6 mice treated with i.p. Aβ + i.n. Aβ [25-fold higher: 1111.6 μg/ml (± 273.1) vs. 44.25 (± 32.5)], i.p. Aβ [17.4-fold higher: 1051.3 μg/ml (± 105.6) vs. 60.6 (± 46.60], i.p. CFA (1st wk) then Aβ nasal [25-fold higher: 24.9 μg/ml (± 26) vs. 0], and i.n. Aβ [7.9-fold higher: 8.1 μg/ml (± 11) vs. 1 (±1.8)]. This difference may be due to strain-specific differences in antigen presentation, B cell activation or complement activation. For both strains, i.p. Aβ, and the combination of i.p. Aβ plus i.n. Aβ led to the highest antibody titers. However, B6D2F1 mice, in particular, generated the highest anti-Aβ antibody titers after receiving the combination treatment.

Serum from Aβ immunized mice was diluted 1:100 and used to immunolabel amyloid-bearing plaques in human AD post-mortem brain sections. Each of six overlapping, 15-residue peptides, spanning the entire Aβ molecule, was incubated individually with serum from Aβ immunized mice. Only the full-length peptide and Aβ1-15 were able to bind the Aβ antibodies in serum, thus preventing plaque staining in AD brain and indicating that the antibodies recognize an epitope(s) within the first 15 amino acids at the N-terminus of Aβ. Biotinylated Ig isotype-specific secondary antibodies were used in conjunction with the mouse serum to immunolabel AD plaques. The anti-Aβ antibodies generated by Aβ immunization were of the IgG1 and IgG2b isotypes, as seen in our first i.n. Aβ immunization study in PDAPP mice.

Use of mucosal adjuvants LT and LT(R192G) for intranasal Aβ immunization

Intranasal vaccines are convenient, well tolerated and cost effective. In our earlier Aβ immunization study, we obtained relatively low titers of Aβ antibodies (~25 μg/ml) in PDAPP mice using i.n. administration of synthetic human Aβ peptide. Using mucosal adjuvants with our i.n. Aβ immunization protocol, we sought to increase the generation of Aβ antibodies in WT mice, in the hopes that higher antibody titers might lead to an even greater reduction of brain Aβ levels in AD mouse models in the future. Mucosal adjuvants have been shown to increase antibody production (both against the antigen and against the adjuvant) and, in some instances, modify the immune response in terms of Ig isotypes and cytokines secreted by antigen-specific T cells (Del Giudice et al. 1999). Mucosal adjuvants induce generation of antigen-specific antibodies both mucosally and systemically. Examples of mucosal adjuvants include bacterial enterotoxins such as cholera toxin (CT) and LT, which are ~80% homologous (Dallas and Falkow 1980). Both have A and B subunits: the A subunit enters the cell, has ADP-ribosyl-transferase enzymatic activity and is considered highly toxic whereas the B subunit binds a receptor and is considered nontoxic (Dickinson and Clements 1995). Cholera toxin B subunit (CTB) and heat-labile toxin (LTB) were used as adjuvants but were less effective than mutant forms of the toxins that are also less toxic (Del Giudice et al. 1999; Dickinson and Clements 1995). Single amino acid substitutions [e.g., LT (R192G)] substantially decrease toxicity by keeping the molecule enzymatically inactive while retaining its strong adjuvanticity (Dickinson and Clements 1995; Chong et al. 1998; Cardenas-Freytag et al. 1999). Mutant LT(R192G) has been evaluated in a number of Phase I and Phase II clinical trials and is safe and non-toxic in humans at adjuvant effective doses (Gluck et al. 1999; Hashigucci et al. 1996).

In our next study, B6D2F1 mice (n = 4 per group) were treated twice a week from 4-12 weeks of age with: 1) 100 μg i.n. Aβ; 2) 100 μg i.n. Aβ + 5 μg LT; 3)100 μg i.n. Aβ + 5 μg LT(R192G); 4) water i.n. + 5 μg LT; 5 water i.n. + 5 μg LT(R192G); or 6) left untreated (Lemere et al. 2002). The Aβ cocktail (three parts Aβ1-40 and one part Aβ1-42; aged O.N. at 37° C) used in the previous study was used here as well. As shown in Figure 1, a significant, 12-fold increase in Aβ antibody titers was detected by ELISA for WT B6D2F1 mice following eight weeks of i.n. immunization with Aβ + LT (285 μg/ml ± 96) compared to Aβ antibody titers from mice treated with i.n. Aβ without adjuvant (23 μg/ml ± 10). The mutant form, LT(R192G), induced an even stronger response; a significant, 16-fold increase in Aβ antibody titer was observed in mice treated with i.n. Aβ + LT(R192G) (376 μg/ml ± 117) compared to titers of mice given i.n. Aβ without adjuvant. In addition, mice treated with i.n. Aβ + LT(R192G) generated antibodies earlier than mice in any of the other treatment groups; Aβ antibodies were evident in two of four mice after only two weeks of treatment and in all four mice after three weeks. Aβ antibody production in mice treated with i.n. Aβ without adjuvant did not begin until the mice had received five weeks of treatment. After eight weeks, these mice produced almost exactly the same level of Aβ antibodies (~23 μg/ml) as in our original study in PDAPP mice, in which no mucosal adjuvant was used. Also in agreement with our earlier data, all Aβ antibodies generated by mice in this study recognized epitope(s) within the first 15 residues of the amino-terminus of Aβ, indicating that this region of Aβ peptide is highly antigenic (Fig. 2). The Aβ antibodies generated in this study were of the following isotypes: IgG1 and IgG2b without adjuvant and included IgG2a and low levels of IgA with adjuvants LT or LT(R192G) (Fig. 3). Both forms of LT were well tolerated by the mice and showed no any obvious toxicity. Mouse brains were examined immunohistochemically. Aβ immunoreactivity was not observed in any of the mouse brains and there were no changes in microglial, astrocytic or tau immunoreactivities in the Aβ immunized mice compared to the vehicle and untreated controls.

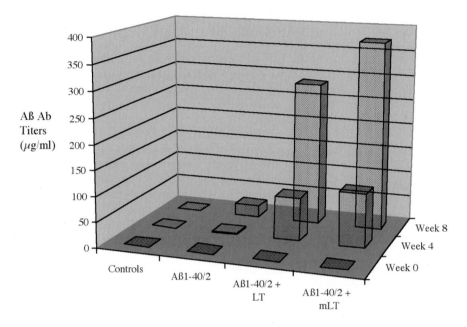

Fig. 1. Anti-Aβ antibody titers were determined by ELISA for the serum of each mouse at each of three time points: pre-immune (Week 0), Week 4 and Week 8. Anti-Aβ antibodies were not detected in any of the pre-immune sera, but their number increased from Week 4 to Week 8 for all groups receiving Aβ . By Week 4, titers were significantly increased in mice immunized with i.n. Aβ + LT(R192G) compared to those of mice treated with i.n. Aβ alone (p < 0.010). By Week 8, Aβ antibody titers in serum from mice treated with i.n. Aβ + LT were increased 12-fold over mice treated with i.n. Aβ alone (p < 0.012). Mutant LT (R192G) led to an even greater increase (16-fold; p < 0.009) in Aβ antibody titers compared to those of mice treated with i.n. Aβ without adjuvant. Higher Aβ antibody titers were achieved using mutant LT(R192G) compared to native LT, in combination with i.n. Aβ, but the difference was not significant. Reprinted from Neurobiology of Aging, Lemere, C. A., Spooner, E. T., Leverone, J. F., Mori, C., and Clements, J. D. Intranasal immunotherapy for the treatment of Alzheimer's disease: *Escherichia coli* LT and LT(R192G) as mucosal adjuvants, 2002 with permission from Elservier Science.

➤

Fig. 2. Aβ antibodies recognized epitopes within the first 15 residues of Aβ, as revealed by the lack of plaque immunoreactivity in serial brain sections from a female AD patient (92 years old) using serum from a B6D2F1 mouse immunized with i.n. Aβ + native LT (Week 8). Absorption of the serum with Aβ1-15 or full-length Aβ peptide abolished plaque immunoreactivity. Absorption of the same serum with five other overlapping 15-mer Aβ peptides, or omission of peptide, allowed detection of plaques by the Aβ antibodies present in the mouse serum, indicating a lack of binding of Aβ antibodies to these regions of Aβ. Scale bar: 100 microns. (Reprinted from Neurobiology of Disease, Lemere, C. A., Spooner, E. T., LaFrancois, J., Malester, B., Mori, C., Leverone, J. F., Matsuoka, Y., Taylor, J. W., DeMattos, R. B., Holtzman, D. M., Clements, J.D., Selkoe, D. J., and Duff, K. E. Evidence for peripheral clearance of cerebral Aβ protein following chronik, aktive Aβ immunization in PSAPP mice, 2003, with permission from Elservier Science).

Epitope-mapping: Nasal Aß40/42 + LT

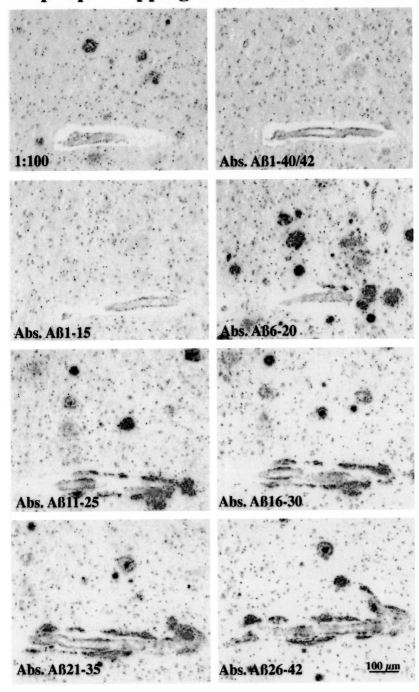

B6D2F1 Sera: Ig Isotyping

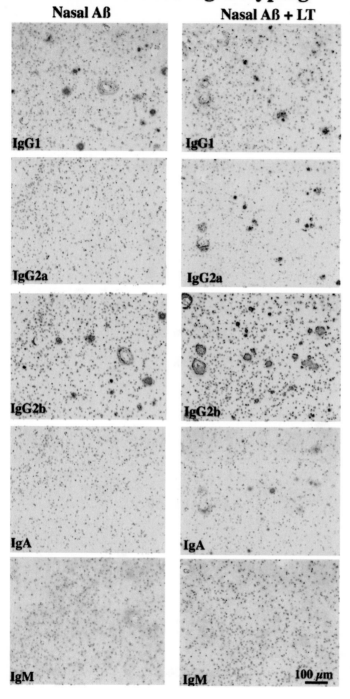

Aβ1-15 as an immunogen for Aβ immunization

In all of our studies, epitope mapping of the Aβ antibodies generated by Aβ immunization revealed that the antibodies recognized a binding site(s) within the first 15 amino acids of the N-terminus of Aβ. Therefore, Aβ1-15 peptide was compared to full-length Aβ for its immunogenicity. B6D2F1 mice (n = 4 per group) were given 100 μg i.n. Aβ1-40/42 or Aβ1-15, each with 10 μg LT(R192G), twice weekly for six weeks (Leverone et al., 2003). Serum from vehicle and untreated control mice lacked Aβ antibodies by ELISA. Generation of Aβ antibodies was evident in mice given i.n. Aβ1-40/42 + LT(R192G) after two to three weeks; Aβ antibody titers were first detected after five weeks of treatment in mice given i.n. Aβ1-15 + LT(R192G). An Aβ antibody ELISA was used to measure Aβ antibody titers. Mice treated with i.n. Aβ1-40/42 + LT(R192G) had very high titers (579 μg/ml ± 196) compared to those of mice treated with i.n. Aβ1-15 + LT(R192G) (16.4 μg/ml ± 18). Again, the antibodies recognized an epitope(s) within the first amino acids of the amino-terminus of Aβ peptide and were of IgG1, IgG2b, IgG2a and IgA isotypes. Aβ, gliosis and neuritic dystrophy were absent from all of the mouse brains.

Aβ immunization of PSAPP mice

In collaboration with Dr. Karen Duff at the Nathan Kline Institute in Orangeburg, NY, we immunized five PSAPP mice by a single i.p. injection of 100 μg of Aβ1-40/42 (CND Biopolymer lab) + 50 μg CFA, and then chronically treated them with i.n. Aβ1-40/42 + 5 μg mucosal adjuvant, LT twice weekly for eight weeks (Lemere et al. 2002, in press). PSAPP mice (Holcomb et al. 1998) were generated by crossing mutant $APP_{K670N,M671L}$ tg mice [Tg2576; (Hsiao et al. 1996)] and mutant $PS1_{M146L}$ mice [line 6.1; (Duff et al. 1996)] and showed accelerated amyloid deposition beginning between 8 and 10 weeks of age. Immunization was started at five weeks of age, prior to plaque formation. Serum Aβ titers from Aβ immunized mice averaged 241 μg/ml, had epitopes within Aβ1-15, and were of IgG1, IgG2b, IgG2a and IgA isotypes as expected. Aβ titers were not detected in serum of vehicle control (n = 2) or untreated control (n = 5) mice. Cerebral Aβ levels were significantly reduced in Aβ immunized mice compared to controls. As depicted in Figure 4, a 75% decrease in plaque number by immunohistochemistry (an aver-

---

Fig. 3. Immunohistochemistry using serum from i.n. Aβ immunized mice and biotinylated Ig isotype-specific secondary antibodies on serial brain sections from a 92-year-old female AD patient showed that, without the use of mucosal adjuvants, Aβ antibodies were predominantly of the immunoglobulin (Ig) isotypes IgG1 and IgG2b (left panel). When LT or LT(R192G) were used as adjuvants for intranasal Aβ immunization, Ig isotypes of the resulting Aβ antibodies included IgG1, IgG2b, IgG2a and a low level of IgA. Plaque immunostaining was not observed using IgM secondary antibodies. Scale bar: 100 microns. (Reprinted from Neurobiology of Aging, Lemere, C. A., Spooner, E. T., Leverone, J. F., Mori, C., and Clements, J. D. Intranasal immunotherapy for the treatment of Alzheimer's disease: *Escherichia coli* LT and LT(R192G) as mucosal adjuvants, 2002 with permission from Elservier Science).

a. Aß plaque immunoreactivity

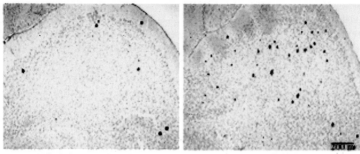

Aß immunized   **Controls**

b.   Plaque counts in PSAPP mouse brain

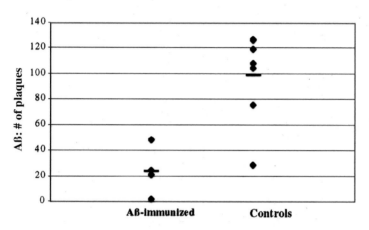

c.   Aßx-42 ELISA: PSAPP brain homogenates

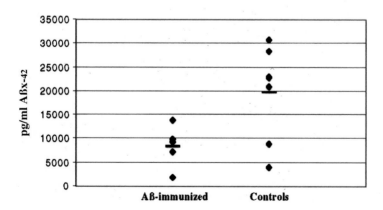

age of 99 plaques vs. 24) was observed as well as a 58% decrease in Aβx-42 by ELISA of guanidine-hydrochloride-extracted brain homogenates (462 pmol/g ± 229 vs. 196 ± 102). Gliosis and neuritic dystrophy were also decreased and corresponded with the remaining compacted Aβ plaques. Vehicle controls showed no abnormal brain pathology, indicating that the adjuvants used in this study, CFA and LT, did not induce an overt inflammatory response in the brain. Kidney, spleen and snout morphologies were indistinguishable in tissues from Aβ immunized mice versus vehicle and untreated controls. Interestingly, a significant, 28-fold increase in serum Aβ1-total was observed in the Aβ immunized mice (52.06 ng/ml ± 23) compared to that of control mice (1.87 ng/ml ± 1.97). In Aβ immunized mice, most of the Aβ protein was bound to Aβ antibodies, as shown by protein G incubation and acid urea gel analysis [protocol provided by Ron DeMattos and David Holtzman (DeMattos et al. 2001)]. Our results are illustrated in Figure 5. Aβ antibodies may clear Aβ from the brain and/or stabilize Aβ in the serum.

Conclusion

In our attempts to further characterize Aβ antibodies and optimize Aβ immunization protocols, we found that WT B6D2F1 mice were more responsive to Aβ immunization than were WT C57BL/6 mice. These data imply that genetic background strains are important for determining the immune response to Aβ vaccination and may be important for interpreting data from Aβ immunization studies in which AD tg mouse models on differing genetic background strains are compared. Intraperitoneal injection of Aβ + adjuvant (CFA/IFA), or a combination treatment of i.p. Aβ (+ CFA/IFA) plus i.n. Aβ (without adjuvant), led to higher anti-Aβ antibody titers than i.n. Aβ alone. A more common protocol for i.p. injections is to give two injections in the first month and then inject monthly. We are currently comparing this schedule of i.p. Aβ immunization with weekly i.n., each with adjuvant, in B6D2F1 mice.

To improve our i.n. Aβ immunization protocol to generate more anti-Aβ antibodies, we employed proven mucosal adjuvants, LT and LT(R192G). Aβ antibody titers were increased 12-fold with LT and 16-fold with LT(R192G) when used with i.n. Aβ in WT mice. High titers of anti-LT antibodies were also observed; however, these seem to have no pathological consequence. Vehicle controls showed no ab-

---

Fig. 4. Cerebral Aß levels in PSAPP mice were reduced following Aß immunization. **a.** Plaques were detected using Aß polyclonal antibody, R1282, for immunohistochemistry on sagittal brain sections from Aß immunized (left) and control (right) PSAPP mice. The presence of discrete, compacted plaques made it feasible to count the plaques in the entire section. **b.** Plaques were counted by visual inspection under the microscope for each of seven sagittal sections at equal planes of section for each mouse. The identity of each mouse was unknown at the time of counting. Aß immunized mice showed a 75% decrease in plaque burden compared to control mice. **c.** Guanidine HCl-extracted cerebral Aß levels were quantified by ELISA. A 58% decrease in Aßx-42 was observed following Aß immunization. (Reprinted from Neurobiology of Aging, Lemere, C. A., Spooner, E. T., Leverone, J. F., Mori, C., and Clements, J. D. Intranasal immunotherapy for the treatment of Alzheimer's disease: *Escherichia coli* LT and LT(R192G) as mucosal adjuvants, 2002 with permission from Elservier Science).

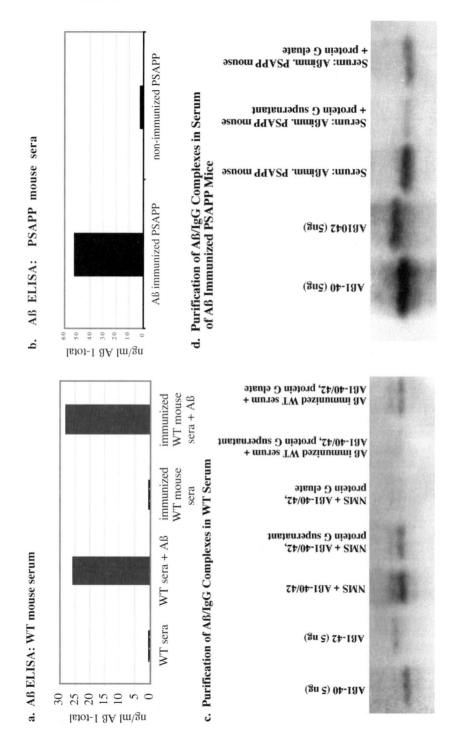

a. Aß ELISA: WT mouse serum

b.   Aß ELISA: PSAPP mouse sera

c. Purification of Aß/IgG Complexes in WT Serum

d. Purification of Aß/IgG Complexes in Serum of Aß Immunized PSAPP Mice

normalities and were indistinguishable from untreated controls. Thus, it appears that LT and, in particular LT(R192G), is very effective at increasing Aβ antibody titers when used with i.n. Aβ immunization in mice and may be effective at inducing Aβ antibody generation in humans when used with i.n. Aβ.

A shorter Aβ peptide, Aβ1-15 was tested for its immunogenicity by giving WT mice the peptide i.n. along with adjuvant, LT(R192G). The results were disappointing; antibody titers were very low. The peptide was completely soluble and never formed aggregates or fibrils. It may be that some sort of aggregate is necessary or beneficial to induce an antibody response, even though data from Sigurdsson et al. (2001) argue that soluble Aβ (1-30 with lysines attached at each end) is an effective immunogen. Degradation of our Aβ1-15 at the mucosal surface, or once transported through the nasal epithelium, is another possible explanation for the lack of immunogenicity. We are currently designing a degradation-resistant Aβ1-15 peptide for i.n. Aβ immunization to answer this question.

Lastly, a prime/boost protocol involving a single i.p. Aβ + CFA injection followed by i.n. Aβ + LT administration twice weekly in PSAPP double tg mice resulted in robust Aβ antibody titers, significantly decreased cerebral Aβ levels, and a corresponding increase in serum Aβ protein levels. These data fit well with the peripheral "sink" hypothesis proposed by DeMattos et al. (2001), which suggests a clearing of CNS Aβ protein to the periphery, and extends it to chronic, active im-

---

Fig. 5. Serum Aβ levels were significantly increased following Aβ immunization in PSAPP mice. **a.** A control experiment was performed to rule out artifactual detection of Aβ in immunized mouse serum. Serum from untreated or Aβ immunized wild type (WT) B6D2F1 was tested by ELISA for the presence of human Aβ before and after spiking with 50 ng Aβ (1:1 ratio of Aβ1-40 and Aβ1-42) in a 500 μl volume. Human Aβ was not detected in untreated or Aβ immunized WT mouse serum. The addition of synthetic human Aβ to serum of untreated or Aβ immunized WT mice allowed detection of Aβ by ELISA; Aβ levels were similar for each mouse and did not vary according to immunization status. **b.** Aβ$_{total}$ ELISA revealed a 28-fold increase in serum Aβ in Aβ immunized vs. untreated PSAPP mice. **c.** Acid/urea step-gradient gel analysis allowed visualization of Aβ. Aβ1-40 (lane 1) and Aβ1-42 (lane 2) were clearly discernible. In a control experiment, Aβ1-40/42 (5 ng each) spiked into WT serum (normal mouse serum, NMS) was detected (lane 3). Protein G beads were added to the mixture to bind antibodies. In the absence of Aβ antibodies in serum from WT untreated mice, Aβ peptide was detected in the supernatant and did not bind to protein G beads (lanes 4 and 5). Serum from Aβ immunized WT mice showed the opposite effect. The spiked Aβ peptide was not observed in the supernatant but instead was eluted from the protein G beads, indicating that the peptide was bound to Aβ antibodies in Aβ immunized mouse serum (lanes 6 and 7). **d.** PSAPP mouse serum was also run on the acid/urea step-gradient gel. A strong Aβ40 band was detected in the mouse serum following denaturation by formic acid (lane 3). Prior to denaturation, serum from an Aβ immunized PSAPP mouse was incubated with anti-mouse IgG and then protein G beads, presumably capturing all antibodies present in the serum. The beads were spun down and the supernatant was exposed to formic acid. Very low levels of Aβ40 were detected in the supernatant. However, when the beads were eluted with formic acid, a distinct, moderately intense Aβ40 band was observed, indicating that the vast majority of Aβ in the serum of Aβ immunized PSAPP mice was bound to antibodies. (Reprinted from Neurobiology of Disease, Lemere, C. A., Spooner, E. T., LaFrancois, J., Malester, B., Mori, C., Leverone, J. F., Matsuoka, Y., Taylor, J. W., DeMattos, R. B., Holtzman, D. M., Clements, J.D., Selkoe, D. J., and Duff, K. E. Evidence for peripheral clearance of cerebral Aβ protein following chronik, aktive Aβ immunization in PSAPP mice, 2003, with permission from Elservier Science).

munization in mice. The increase in serum Aβ was 28-fold here, as opposed to 1000-fold in their earlier study, but several points may explain the difference. First, our mice were actively immunized over an eight-week period, as opposed to being given passive transfer of an Aβ monoclonal antibody by intravenous injection and then measuring peripheral Aβ several days later. Both studies showed binding of Aβ to antibodies in the blood. Presumably, these complexes would be cleared over time, resulting in lower Aβ levels in the periphery. We are currently examining spleen, liver and kidney tissues from Aβ immunized PSAPP mice to determine the pathway of clearance of these antibody/antigen complexes. Second, we measured Aβ in serum; they measured it in plasma. Some Aβ may have been spun down in the purification of serum from blood. Third, differences in AD tg mouse models, ages, and Aβ vaccination protocols may also account for some of the differences in absolute levels of Aβ. Our results are consistent with a mechanism whereby the efflux of soluble Aβ from the brain to the periphery, leading to increased levels of Aβ/anti-Aβ antibody complexes in the blood, appears to play a role in the lowering of cerebral Aβ following Aβ immunization. Sequestering Aβ from the brain to the blood may be an effective therapeutic strategy for the prevention and/or treatment of AD in humans.

Acknowledgments

We thank Drs. Karen Duff, Dennis Selkoe, Ronald DeMattos and David Holtzman for their contributions to these studies. Funding was provided, in part, by the Alzheimer's Association (IIRG to CAL) and the National Institute of Aging (RO1 to CAL).

Reference

Bacskai BJ, Kajdasz ST, Christie RH, Carter C, Games D, Seubert P, Schenk D, Hyman BT (2001) Imaging of amyloid-β deposits in brains of living mice permits direct observation of clearance of plaques with immunotherapy. Nature Med. 7:369–372.
Bard F, Cannon C, Barbour R, Burke RL, Games D, Grajeda H, Guido T, Hu K, Huang J, Johnson-Wood K, Khan K, Kholodenko D, Lee M, Lieberburg I, Motter R, Nguyen M, Soriano F, Vasquez N, Weiss K, Welch B, Seubert P, Schenk D, Yednock T (2000) Peripherally administered antibodies against amyloid beta-peptide enter the central nervous system and reduce pathology in a mouse model of Alzheimer disease. Nature Med 6:916–919.
Brayden D, Templeton L, McClean S, Barbour R, Huang J, Nguyen M, Ahern D, Motter R, Johnson-Wood K, Vasquez N, Schenk D, Seubert P (2001) Encapsulation in biodegradable microparticles enhances serum antibody response to parenterally-delivered β-amyloid in mice. Vaccine 19:4185–4193.
Cardenas-Freytag L, Cheng E, Mayeux P, Domer JE, Clements JD (1999) Effectiveness of a vaccine composed of heat-killed Candida albicans and a novel mucosal adjuvant, LT(R192G), against systemic candidiasis. Infect Immunol 67:826–833.
Chong CM, Friberg M, Clements JD (1998) LT(R192G), a non-toxic mutant of the heat-labile enterotoxin of Esherichia coli, elicits enhanced humoral and cellular immune responses associated with protection against lethal oral challenge with Salmonella spp. Vaccine 16:732–740.

Dallas WS, Falkow S (1980) Amino acid sequence homology between cholera toxin and Escherichia coli heat-labile toxin. Nature 288:499–501.

Del Giudice G, Pizza M, Rappuoli R (1999) Mucosal delivery of vaccines. Methods 19:148–155.

DeMattos RB, Bales KR, Cummins DJ, Dodart J-C, Paul SM, Holtzman DM (2001) Peripheral anti-Aβ antibody alters CND and plasma clearance and decreases brain Aβ burden in a mouse model of Alzheimer's disease. Proc Natl Acad Sci USA 98:8850–8855.

Dickinson BL, Clements JD (1995) Dissociation of Escherichia coli heat-labile enterotoxin adjuvanticity from ADP-ribosyltransferase activity. Infect Immunol 63:1617–1623.

Duff K, Eckman C, Zehr C, Yu X, Prada C-M, Perez-Tur J, Hutton M, Buee L, Harigaya Y, Yager D, Morgan D, Gordon MN, Holcomb L, Refolo L, Zenk B, Hardy J, Younkin S (1996) Increased amyloid-β42(43) in brains of mice expressing mutant presenilin 1. Nature 383:710–713.

Frenkel D, Katz O, Solomon B (2000) Immunization against Alzheimer's β-amyloid plaques via EFRH phage administration. Proc Natl Acad Sci USA 97:11455–11459.

Gluck U, Gebbers J-O, Gluck R (1999) Phase 1 evaluation of intranasal virosomal influenza vaccine with and without Escherichia coli heat-labile toxin in adult volunteers. J Virol 73:7780–7786.

Hashigucci K, Ogawa H, Ishidate T, Yamashita R, Kamiya H, Watanabe K, Hattori N, Sato T, Suzuki Y, Nagamine T, Aizawa C, Tamura S, Kurata T, Oya A (1996) Antibody responses in volunteers induced by nasal influenza vaccine combined with Escherichia coli heat-labile enterotoxin B subunit containing trace amount of the holotoxin. Vaccine 14:113–119.

Holcomb L, Gordon MN, McGowan E, Yu X, Benkovic S, Jantzen P, Wright K, Saad I, Mueller R, Morgan D, Sanders S, Zehr C, O'Campo K, Hardy J, Prada CM, Eckman C, Younkin S, Hsiao K, Duff K (1998) Accelerated Alzheimer-type phenotype in transgenic mice carrying both mutant amyloid precursor protein and presenilin 1 transgenes. Nature Med 4:97–100.

Hsiao K, Chapman P, Nilsen S, Ekman C, Harigaya Y, Younkin S, Yang F, Cole G (1996) Correlative memory deficits, Aβ elevation, and amyloid plaques in transgenic mice. Science 274:99–102.

Janus C, Pearson J, McLaurin J, Mathews PM, Jiang Y, Schmidt SD, Chishti MA, Horne P, Heslin D, French J, Mount HT, Nixon RA, Mercken M, Bergeron C, Fraser PE, St George-Hyslop P, Westaway D (2000) A beta peptide immunization reduces behavioural impairment and plaques in a model of Alzheimer's disease. Nature 408:979–982.

Lemere CA, Maron R, Spooner ET, Grenfell TJ, Mori C, Desai R, Hancock WW, Weiner HL, Selkoe DJ (2000) Nasal Aβ treatment induces anti-Aβ antibody production and decreases cerebral amyloid burden in PD-APP mice. Ann N Y Acad Sci. 920:328–331.

Lemere CA, Spooner ET, Leverone JF, Mori C, Clements JD (2002) Intranasal immunotherapy for the treatment of Alzheimer's disease: Escherichia coli LT and LT(R192G) as mucosal adjuvants. Neurobiol Aging, 23:991–1000.

Lemere CA, Spooner ET, LaFrancois J, Malester B, Mori C, Leverone JF, Matsuoka Y, Taylor JW, De Mattos RB, Holtzman DM, Clements JD, Selkoe DJ, Duff KE (2003) Evidence for peripheral clearance of cerebral Aβ protein following chronic, active Aβ immunization in PSAPP mice. Neurobiol Dis, in press.

Leverone JF, Spooner ET, Lehmann H, Clements JD, Lemere CA (2002; in press online 23 Dec, 2002) Aβ1-15 in less unnzbigebuc tgab Aβ1-40/42 for intranasal immunization of wild-type mice but may be effective for boosting. Vaccine, in press.

Morgan D, Diamond DM, Gottschall PE, Ugen KE, Dickey C, Hardy J, Duff K, Jantzen P, DiCarlo G, Wilcock D, Connor K, Hatcher J, Hope C, Gordon M, Arendash GW (2000) A beta peptide vaccination prevents memory loss in an animal model of Alzheimer's disease. Nature 408:982–985.

Morokata T, Ishikawa J, Ida K, Yamada T (1999) C57BL/6 mice are more susceptible to antigen-induced pulmonary eosinophilia than BALB/c mice, irrespective of systemic T helper 1/T helper responses. Immunology 98:345–351.

Schenk D, Barbour R, Dunn W, Gordon G, Grajeda H, Guido T, Hu K, Huang J, Johnson-Wood K, Khan K, Kholodenko D, Lee M, Liao Z, Lieberburg I, Motter R, Mutter L, Soriano F, Shopp G, Vasquez N, Vendevert C, Walker S, Wogulis M, Yednock T, Games D, Seubert P (1999) Immunization with amyloid-β attenuates Alzheimer-disease-like pathology in the PDAPP mouse. Nature 400:173–177.

Selkoe DJ (1999) Translating cell biology into therapeutic advances in Alzheimer's disease. Nature 399:A23–A31.

Sigurdsson EM, Scholtzova H, Mehta PD, Frangione B, Wisniewski T (2001) Immunization with a non-toxic/non-fibrillar amyloid-β homologous peptide reduces Alzheimer's disease-associated pathology in transgenic mice. Am J Pathol 159:439–447.

Spooner ET, Desai RV, Mori C, Leverone JF, Lemere CA (2002) The generation and characteriuation of ptentially therapeutic Aβ antibodies in mice: differences according to strain and immunization protocol. Vaccine 21:290–297.

Weiner HL, Lemere CA, Maron R, Spooner ET, Grenfell TJ, Mori C, Issazadeh S, Hancock WW, Selkoe DJ (2000) Nasal administration of amyloid-beta peptide decreases cerebral amyloid burden in a mouse model of Alzheimer's disease. Ann Neurol 48:567–579.

Antibody Therapy Against β-Amyloid to Treat Alzheimer's Disease

F. Bard, P. Seubert, D. Schenk, and T. Yednock

Summary

In transgenic mouse models of Alzheimer's disease (AD), immunization with beta-amyloid peptide Aβ1-42 slows or reverses disease progression and provides neuronal protection and improvement in memory tasks. Development of a safe and effective immunization strategy for therapeutic use requires an understanding of the immune system components involved in these responses. A key discovery has been that reduction of AD-like neuropathologies can be obtained with passive administration of antibodies, and that a T cell response against Aβ is not required. Several mechanisms have been suggested to be involved in efficacy, including antibody Fc-mediated and Fc-independent events; these mechanisms are reviewed here.

Introduction

One of the defining neuropathological characteristics of Alzheimer's disease (AD) is the extracellular accumulation and deposition of the beta-amyloid peptide (Aβ) within plaques (Glenner and Wong 1984). The predominant component of these plaques is a 42amino acid-long isoform ($Aβ_{42}$) that is prone to aggregation. There is mounting evidence that plaques and/or other aggregated forms of Aβ play an important role in neuronal dysfunction and the development of cognitive deficits (Selkoe 2000; Sisodia 1999; St George-Hyslop 1999). Consequently, various approaches are being developed with the aim of reducing Aβ levels in the brain for the treatment of AD (reviewed in Schenk et al. 2001). A critical tool in these studies has been a transgenic mouse strain that overexpresses disease-linked isoforms of the human amyloid precursor protein (APP) and shows hallmark features of AD, including Aβ deposition in plaques, neuronal dystrophy, synaptic loss, and cognitive deficits.

Several investigators have shown that immunization of APP transgenic mice with $Aβ_{42}$ improves neuropathological and behavioral outcomes (Schenk et al. 1999; Morgan et al. 2000; Janus et al. 2000). A detailed understanding of the immune components required for efficacy is necessary to derive the best therapeutic

Elan Pharmaceuticals, 800 Gateway Blvd, South San Francisco, CA 94080, USA

Selkoe/Christen
Immunization Against Alzheimer's Disease
and Other Neurodegenerative Disorders
© Springer-Verlag Berlin Heidelberg 2003

approach based on these findings. Several lines of evidence indicate that an antibody response, rather than a cellular immune response, is key to immunotherapeutic benefit in APP mice. Most importantly, passive administration of antibodies against Aβ is sufficient to prevent plaque deposition, induce plaque clearance, and protect against neuronal damage. Indeed, antibodies directed against the N-terminus of Aβ can bind to amyloid plaques and induce Fc-mediated clearance through the actions of microglial cells, both in vivo and ex vivo (Bard et al. 2000). However, it has been reported that a degree of antibody-mediated efficacy can also be obtained by mechanisms that are independent of Fc interactions. One study indicated that an antibody that is directed against the mid-portion of soluble Aβ, and which cannot recognize plaques, appears to reduce plaque deposition (DeMattos et al. 2001). It has also been suggested that antibodies against a particular epitope on Aβ (EFRH) can cause disaggregation of the peptide in vitro and perhaps lead to plaque dissolution (Solomon et al. 1996, 1997; Frenkel et al. 1999). These and other potential mechanisms of efficacy will be discussed in this review.

Fc Receptor-Mediated Clearance of Aβ by Microglial Cells

Antibodies enter the central nervous system (CNS) at low but significant levels. Under normal circumstances, brain levels of antibody are approximately 0.1% the levels in the blood, regardless of antibody isotype (Ganrot and Laurell 1974; Bard et al., unpublished data). Thus antibodies against the amino terminus of Aβ, even when administered via intravenous injection, passively enter the CNS and accumulate on plaques. Notably, microglial cells containing amyloid peptide are commonly found in the vicinity of plaques following either Aβ immunization (Schenk et al. 1999) or passive administration of anti-Aβ antibodies that induced amyloid plaque clearance. Such Aβ-positive cells are only rarely observed in brain tissue from patients with AD and have never been seen in tissue from non-immunized APP mice (Stadler et al. 2001). These results suggest that anti-Aβ antibodies are able to coat amyloid plaques and trigger microglial phagocytosis and plaque clearance. Consistent with this idea, Fc-dependent, antibody-mediated phagocytosis of plaques can be measured in an ex vivo assay in brain tissue from patients with AD or from APP transgenic mice (Bard et al. 2000). In the presence of antibodies directed against Aβ, microglial cells are able to clear plaques in unfixed sections of brain tissue within 24 hours. In contrast, in sections incubated in the absence of antibody, or in those incubated with antibodies lacking intact Fc regions, microglial cells do not appear to interact with plaques, and microglial clearance of amyloid is not observed. Moreover, microglial cells lacking functional Fc receptors are unable to clear plaques even in the presence of intact antibodies (Bard et al., unpublished). This assay is important since it has proven to be predictive of in vivo efficacy in reducing the progression of AD-like neuropathologies. Specifically, antibodies against Aβ that fail to trigger phagocytosis of plaques in the ex vivo assay are also comparatively inactive towards reducing neuropathology in vivo. The assay predicts, and in vivo results confirm, that antibodies directed against epitopes within the first 7 to 10 amino acids of Aβ provide the greatest degree of efficacy in reducing plaque-associated neuropathologies.

Fc-receptor-mediated uptake of Aβ in the ex vivo assay leads to rapid degradation of the peptide, whereas Aβ is degraded very slowly following uptake through other pathways, such as those mediated by different types of scavenger receptors (Paresce et al. 1996). It appears that Fc-induced phagosomes are lead through a lysosomal pathway with different catabolic activity than the non-Fc phagosomes (Claus et al. 1998). It is interesting to note that microglial cells have a different phagocytotic activity for synthetic Aβ than for Aβ in amyloid plaques. Synthetic Aβ is readily phagocytosed, whereas phagocytosis of Aβ within amyloid plaques does not occur in the absence of antibodies (Ard et al. 1996; Bard et al., unpublished observations). Furthermore, unlike our observations with Aβ in plaques, Brazil et al. (2000) found that antibodies did not affect the slow degradation rate of synthetic fibrillar Aβ.

In a study that we presented at the Ipsen meeting in March 2002, plaque-bearing PDAPP mice were immunized with small fragments of Aβ peptide linked to a T cell epitope derived from an unrelated antigen. The fragments included Aβ1-5, Aβ3-9, Aβ5-11, and Aβ15-24, and each generated a comparable antibody response as measured by reactivity with synthetic, aggregated Aβ1-42. Sera from all mice immunized with the three N-terminal peptides (Aβ1-5, Aβ3-9, and Aβ5-11) were able to react with plaques in unfixed brain sections. Furthermore, mice immunized with these peptides had reduced plaque burden and significantly reduced neuronal damage, as measured by reduction of neuritic burden, compared to control immunized mice. Although there was a strong antibody response against Aβ15-24, and sera from all mice immunized with this peptide could react with synthetic Aβ, none of the sera could bind to Aβ within plaques. Likewise, these mice were not protected against plaque deposition and neuronal dystrophy. These results strongly support an important role for Fc-mediated plaque clearance in protection against neuronal damage. Other mechanisms whereby anti-Aβ antibodies may be beneficial are possible, however, as discussed below.

Fc-Dependent, Complement-Mediated Clearance

Upon antibody binding to its cognate antigen, one function of the antibody Fc region is to activate the complement cascade, which results in covalent modification of the antigen with the complement components C3bi and C3d. These modifications are then recognized by specific complement receptors expressed on phagocytotic cells (CR3 and CR4 for C3bi; CR1 and CR2 for C3d). The role of complement in amyloid clearance in the immunization paradigm has not yet been addressed. In the ex vivo assay, microglial cells would need to provide complement themselves since the assay can be successfully performed in medium lacking exogenous complement components. However, complement alone appears to be insufficient for plaque clearance, since phagocytosis is prevented by inhibition of Fc receptor interactions, as discussed above. Also, amyloid burden reduction is obtained with an antibody against Aβ of the IgG1 isotype, which does not bind complement (Bard et al. 2000 and see below). These results do not eliminate a potential contribution of complement in vivo. In other in vivo systems, complement and Fc receptors on phagocytic cells may work together to provide a clearance response, although complement activation requires a higher concentration of antibody, with a higher density of target opsonization, than is required for Fc-mediated phagocytosis (Azeredo da Silveira et al. 2002). Interestingly, immunization of seven- to eight-month-old APP transgenic mice crossed with FcR- deficient mice lead to reduced Aβ levels in the brain (Das et al. 2001), suggesting either a non-Fc-mediated mechanism or a potential role for complement in amyloid clearance. In vitro, fibrillar Aβ can itself activate complement through an alternative pathway (Webster et al. 2001) and complement may be part of the normal pathway for Aβ clearance in vivo (Wyss-Coray et al. 2001, 2002). This process could be augmented by antibody opsonization of the peptide. Further studies are required to fully address the role of complement in amyloid clearance.

If Fc-dependent interactions are important for plaque clearance and/or neuronal protection, then the isotype of the antibody response should affect the degree of efficacy. In our presentation at the Ipsen meeting in March 2002, we also discussed a study in which we compared six monoclonal antibodies directed against the same epitope of Aβ peptide (Aβ1-7) but of different isotypes; two were IgG1, two were IgG2a, and two were IgG2b. Murine IgG2a exhibits the highest affinity for Fc receptors involved in phagocytosis and efficiently activates complement. IgG2b also activates complement but exhibits a somewhat lower affinity for murine Fc receptors. IgG1 cannot fix complement, and although it binds to the Fc receptors with low affinity, it can still effectively trigger Fc receptor-mediated phagocytosis of opsonized antigen (Azeredo da Silveira et al. 2002). All of the antibodies were administered weekly to APP transgenic mice at a dose of 10 mg/kg/week for six months and maintained equivalent titers throughout the course of the study. Among the six antibodies, the IgG2a antibodies exhibited the lowest avidity for deposited Aβ. In addition, one of these antibodies was unable to capture soluble Aβ, while the other exhibited moderate capture ability. In spite of these limitations, the two IgG2a antibodies provided the highest degree of plaque clearance and were the only two antibodies to provide significant protection against neuronal damage. These findings are important because they demonstrate that passively administered antibodies can protect neurons against damage in APP transgenic mice, and they support the hypothesis that antibody Fc effector functions play an important role in efficacy.

Non-Fc-Mediated Amyloid Clearance

Using multiphoton microscopy, a novel technique for in vivo imaging of amyloid plaques in transgenic APP mice, Bacskai et al. (2001a) demonstrated that deposition of both diffuse and fibrillar amyloid was reversed by direct application of an anti-Aβ antibody to the cerebral cortex. The application, involving a high concentration of antibody solution (1 mg/ml), induced clearance of amyloid plaques within three days. An increased microglial response around the remaining amyloid deposits at the treatment site was also observed, whereas there were few microglia associated with plaques distal to the site of injection. These results are similar to those obtained with the ex vivo assay and support the role of antibodies and microglial cells in mediating plaque clearance. However, using the same technique, this group has recently shown that anti-Aβ antibody fragments lacking the Fc region (Fab'2) also lead to clearance of amyloid deposits within three days of administration (Bacskai et al. 2001b). If a dynamic equilibrium exists between deposited and soluble Aβ, it is possible that an antibody directed against Aβ could shift the equilibrium in favor of the soluble form – a process that could occur through antibody/antigen interactions independent of the Fc domain. Although the concentrations of antibody applied to the brain in these studies were much higher than could be achieved in the CNS through peripheral administration, it may be possible to affect the equilibrium of Aβ at lower antibody levels (see below). To better understand this process, it will be important to determine the antibody concentration required for efficacy and to investigate whether an increased microglial response was associated with plaque clearance following Fab'2 application.

Disaggregation of Amyloid Fibrils

It has also been suggested that antibodies against Aβ can directly prevent and even reverse the formation of amyloid fibrils (Solomon et al. 1996, 1997). A one-to-one molar ratio of antibody to Aβ is required for fibril dissolution in vitro; however, it is possible that a more dynamic equilibrium between deposited and soluble Aβ exists in vivo than in vitro, allowing for a significant clearance response at the low antibody levels observed in the brain with peripheral immunization. Also, lower in vitro concentrations of antibody appear to be sufficient for prevention, rather than reversal, of Aβ fibril formation, suggesting that prevention of plaque deposition could be a more important mechanism with low CNS antibody levels. Antibodies that have been shown to inhibit or reverse Aβ fibrillarization have high affinity specificity for the sequence EFRH corresponding to position 3-7 of the Aβ peptide (Frenkel et al. 1999). However, since antibodies against Aβ1-5, are also effective in vivo, a broader region of the N-terminus may be involved in fibrillarization or other mechanisms of clearance could be involved.

"Peripheral Aβ Sink" by Anti- Aβ Antibodies

An additional mechanism for the clearance of Aβ has recently been proposed based on in vivo studies with passive administration of the murine antibody 266 (DeMattos et al. 2001). This antibody fails to bind amyloid plaques and does not work in the ex vivo assay (Bard et al., unpublished), but binds avidly to soluble Aβ. Within a few days of intravenous injection of antibody 266, total Aβ plasma levels (found to be complexed with the antibody) were increased by 1000-fold. A five-month treatment of young mice with antibody 266, before the onset of plaque deposition, reduced Aβ levels in the cortex. It was proposed that antibodies bind to Aβ peptide in the periphery and prevent their re-entry into the CNS. The peripheral sink would thus alter the equilibrium between blood and brain levels of Aβ. However, this interpretation of the data is complicated by the fact that the majority of Aβ in PDAPP transgenic mice is produced within the CNS, and its half-life in plasma is only minutes. In young mice prior to plaque deposition, brain levels of Aβ are approximately 10-fold higher than those in plasma and become even higher as Aβ deposits in the brain with age. Thus, it is difficult to explain why stabilization of circulating plasma Aβ with antibody 266 would significantly decrease brain levels of the peptide.

An alternative explanation of the data is that antibody 266 passively enters the CNS at low levels (as with other antibodies described above), binds to soluble Aβ, and reduces deposition of plaques. Consistent with this idea, a subsequent publication (Dodart et al. 2002) showed that reversal of memory deficits, as measured in an object recognition task and a holeboard learning and memory task, was observed only when antibody 266/Aβ complexes could be observed in the CNS. Remarkably, it was also shown that treatment with the antibody at doses greater than 10mg/kg caused behavioral improvement in PDAPP mice within 24 hours of administration. A similar degree of improvement was observed 24 hours after one dose or 72 hours after the last of five weekly doses. At these doses and time points, the concentration of antibody 266 in the CNS is likely to have been greater than 100 ng/ml (0.67 nM), which is close to the IC_{50} of the antibody for capture of soluble Aβ (2 nM; P. Seubert, personal communication). These results suggest that the antibody binds to Aβ or soluble aggregates in a stoichiometric fashion to inhibit at least some of the direct effects that Aβ may have on neurons (Walsh et al. 2002). The interplay between soluble Aβ, plaques, and neuronal damage is unknown but can be elucidated by studies with antibodies such as 266 and those described above with different Aβ-binding properties.

Therapeutic Opportunities

The discovery that antibodies against Aβ peptide can enter the brain and protect neurons against pathologic changes associated with AD has opened a number of potential therapeutic opportunities. As shown in Table 1, at least four different antibody-based approaches can be envisioned, each engaging different aspects of the immune system. The most straightforward approach would be immunization with Aβ peptide itself, where T cells and B cells are activated against Aβ and collaborate in the production of antibodies. The antibodies against Aβ can then passively enter the CNS to protect neurons in a variety of ways, including the activation of an Aβ clearance response by microglial cells. A potential drawback of this approach is that T cells directed against Aβ, a self-peptide enriched in the brain, could be deleterious. Recent clinical evidence found that ~5% of AD patients receiving Aβ1-42 immunizations developed encephalitis, suggesting that this may occur in a subset of patients. Since a T cell response directed against Aβ peptide is not necessary for efficacy, an alternative immunization strategy could involve constructs that present key antibody epitopes derived from Aβ in conjunction with foreign T cell epitopes. As described above, a variety of such constructs has been shown to be effective in APP transgenic mice. Finally, it is possible to develop recombinant human antibodies against specific epitopes of Aβ for antibody

Table 1. Immunization against Alzheimer's disease: The divesity of therapeutic opportunities.

Therapeutic approach	Immune cell involvement			
	T cells	B cells	Microglia	Passive clearance
Immunization with Aβ peptide	+	+	+	+
Immunization with construct containing Aβ antibody epitope	–	+	+	+
Treatment with a human antibody against Aβ, optimized for clearance by microglial cells thru Fc interaction	–	–	+	+
Treatment with a human antibody optimized for passive clearance	–	–	–	+

therapy – thereby eliminating the need to activate a B cell response, which may be difficult to achieve in all patients. The antibodies can be designed to trigger Fc-mediated clearance by microglial cells, to disrupt plaque deposition independent of microglial cells, and/or to directly block effects of Aβ on neurons.

Our data suggest that Fc-mediated clearance of Aβ peptide by microglial cells is a highly efficient and therapeutically effective approach in reducing AD-like neuropathology in mice, since 1) Fc interactions appear to be key for clearance of plaques in an ex vivo assay; 2) there is an excellent correlation between antibodies that are effective in the ex vivo assay and those that are neuroprotective in APP transgenic mice; and 3) when comparing a number of parameters among antibodies against Aβ, the isotype of the Fc domain plays an important role. Mouse IgG2a antibodies, which exhibit the highest level of Fc effector function, provide the highest degree of efficacy, as defined by plaque clearance, protection against neuronal dystrophy, and protection against synaptic loss. The therapeutic opportunities described in Table 1 cover a range of approaches and, because of the importance of developing a disease-modifying therapy for AD, it will be critical to determine the clinical utility of these approaches.

References

Ard MD, Cole GM, Wei J. Mehrle AP, Fratkin JD (1996) Scavenging of Alzheimer's amyloid β-protein by microglia in culture. J Neurosci Res 43:190–202

Azeredo da Silveira S, Kikuchi S, Fossati-Jimack L, Moll T, Saito T, Verbeek JS, Botto M, Walport MJ, Carroll M, Izui S (2002) Complement activation selectively potentiates the pathogenicity of the IgG2b and IgG3 isotypes of a high affinity anti-erythrocyte autoantibody. J Exp Med 195(6):665–672

Bacskai BJ, Kajdasz ST, Christie RH, Carter C, Games D, Seubert P, Schenk D, Hyman BT (2001a) Imaging of beta-amyloid deposits in brains of living mice permits direct observation of clearance of plaques with immunotherapy. Nature Med 7:369–372

Bacskai BJ, Kajdasz ST, McLellan ME, Games D, Seubert P, Schenk D, Hyman BT (2001b) Multiple mechanisms are involved in clearance of amyloid-β by immunotherapy. Soc Neurosci Abstr 27#687.7

Bard F, Cannon, C Barbour R, RL, Burke RL Games D, Grajeda H, Guido T, Hu K, Huang J, John-son-Wood K, Khan K, Kholodenko D, Lee M, Lieberburg I, Motter R, Nguyen M, Soriano F, Vasquez N, Weiss K, Welch B, Seubert P, Schenk D, Yednock T (2000) Peripherally administered antibodies against amyloid beta-peptide enter the central nervous system and reduce pathology in a mouse model of Alzheimer disease. Nature Med 6:916–919

Brazil MI, Chung H, Maxfield FR (2000) Effects of incorporation of immunoglobulin G and complement component C1q on uptake and degradation of Alzheimer's disease amyloid fibrils by microglia. J Biol Chem 2759220:16941–16947

Claus V, Jahraus A, Tjelle T, Berg T, Kirschke H, Faulstich H, Griffiths G (1998) Lysosomal enzyme trafficking between phagosomes, endosomes, and lysosomes in J774 macrophages. J Biol Chem 273 (16):9842–9851

Das P, Murphy MP, Loosbrock N, Smith TE, Nicolle M, and Golde TE (2001) Further studies on abeta immunization in TG2576 mice: effects of pre-existing amyloid deposition and Fc receptor knockout. Soc Neurosci Abstr 27# 649.3

DeMattos RB, Bales KR, Cummins DJ, Dodart JC, Paul SM, Holtzman DM (2001) Peripheral anti-Aβ antibody alters CNS and plasma Aβ clearance and decreases brain Aβ burden in a mouse model of Alzheimer's disease. Proc.Natl.Acad.Sci. USA 98:8850–8855

Dodart JC, Bales KR, Gannon KS, Greene SJ, DeMattos RB, Mathis C, DeLong CA, Wu S, Wu X, Holtzman DM, Paul S (2002) Immunization reverses memory deficits without reducing brain Aβ burden in Alzheimer's disease model. Nature Neurosci 5(5):452–457

Frenkel D, Balass M, Katchalski-Katzir E, Solomon B (1999) High affinity binding of monoclonal antibodies to the sequential epitope EFRH of beta-amyloid peptide is essential for modulation of fibrillar aggregation. J Neuroimmunol 95 (1-2):136–142

Ganrot K, Laurell C-B (1974) Measurement of IgG and albumin content of cerebrospinal fluid, and its interpretation. Clin Chem 20:571–573

Glenner GC, Wong CW (1984) Alzheimer's disease: initial report of the purification and characterization of a novel cerebrovascular amyloid protein. Biochem Biophys Res Commun 120:855–890

Janus C, Pearson J, McLaurin J, Mathews PM, Jiang Y, Schmidt SD, Chishti MA, Horne P, Heslin D, French J, Mount HT, Nixon RA, Mercken M, Bergeron C, Fraser PE, St George-Hyslop P, Westaway D (2000) A beta peptide immunization reduces behavioural impairment and plaques in a model of Alzheimer's disease. Nature 408:979–982

Morgan D, Diamond DM, Gottschall PE, Ugen KE, Dickey C, Hardy J, Duff K, Jantzen P, DiCarlo G, Wilcock D, Connor K, Hatcher J, Hope C, Gordon M, Arendash GW (2000) A beta peptide vaccination prevents memory loss in an animal model of Alzheimer's disease. Nature 408:982–985

Paresce DM, Ghosh RN, Maxfield FR (1996) Microglial cells internalize aggregates of the Alzheimer's disease amyloid β-protein via a scavenger receptor. Neuron 17:553–565

Schenk D, Barbour R, Dunn W, Gordon G, Grajeda H, Guido T, Hu K, Huang J, Johnson-Wood K, Khan K, Kholodenko D, Lee M, Liao Z, Lieberburg I, Motter R, Mutter L, Soriano F, Shopp G, Vasquez N, Vandevert C, Walker S, Wogulis M, Yednock T, Games G, Seubert P (1999) Immunization with amyloid-beta attenuates Alzheimer-disease-like pathology in the PDAPP mouse. Nature 400:173–177

Schenk D, Games D, Seubert P (2001) Potential treatment opportunities for Alzheimer's disease through inhibition of secretases and Aβ immunization. J Mol Neuro 17:259–267

Selkoe DJ (2000) The genetics and molecular pathology of Alzheimer's disease: roles of amyloid and the presenilins. Neurol Clin 18:903–922

Sisodia SS (1999) Alzheimer's disease:perspectives for the new millenium. J Clin Invest 104:1169–1170

Solomon B, Koppel R, Hanan E, Katzav T (1996) Monoclonal antibodies inhibit *in vitro* fibrillar aggregation of the Alzheimer β-amyloid peptide. Proc Natl Acad Sci 93:452–455

Solomon B, Koppel R, Frankel D, Hanan-Aharon E (1997) Disaggregation of Alzheimer β-amyloid by site-directed mAb. Proc Natl Acad Sci 94:4109–4112

Stadler M, Deller T, Staufenbiel M, Jucker M (2001) 3D-reconstruction of microglia and amyloid in APP23 transgenic mice: no evidence of intracellular amyloid. Neurobiol Aging 22(3):427–434

St. George-Hyslop PH (1999) Molecular genetics of Alzheimer disease. Sem Neurol 19:371–383

Walsh DM, Klyubin I, Fadeeva JV, Cullen WK, Anwyl R, Wolfe MS, Rowan MJ, Selkoe DJ (2002) Naturally secreted oligomers of amyloid β protein potently inhibit hippocampal long-term potentiation *in vivo*. Nature 416:535–539

Webster SD, Galvan MD, Ferran E, Garzon-Rodriguez, Glabe CG, Tenner AJ (2001) Antibody-mediated phagocytosis of the amyloid β-peptide in microglia is differentially modulated by C1q. J. Immunology 166:7496–7503

Wyss-Coray T, Lin AH, Alexander JJ, Quigg RJ, Yan F (2001) Genetic inhibition of the complement cascade increases Alzheimer's pathology in transgenic mice. Soc Neurosci Abstr 27:687.4

Wyss-Coray T, Yan F, Hsiu-Ti Lin A, Lambris JD, Alexander JJ, Quigg RL, Masliah E (2002) Prominent neurodegeneration and increased plaque formation in complement inhibited Alzheimer's mice. Proc Natl Acad Sci 99:10837–10842

Effects of a Peripheral Anti-Aβ Antibody on Plasma and CNS Aβ Clearance

D. M. Holtzman[1,2,3,4], K. R. Bales[5], S. M. Paul[5], R. B. DeMattos[1,2,3]

Summary

Active immunization with the amyloid-β (Aβ) peptide has been shown to decrease brain Aβ deposition in transgenic mouse models of Alzheimer's disease (AD), and certain peripherally administered anti-Aβ antibodies mimic this effect. The mechanism(s) underlying these effects is under investigation. PDAPP mice represent a transgenic mouse model of AD. Interestingly, in young PDAPP mice that lack AD pathology, levels of CSF and plasma Aβ are strongly correlated and thus appear to be in equilibrium. In contrast, this correlation is absent in older PDAPP mice with plaques. We explored whether the presence in the periphery of a monoclonal anti-Aβ antibody (m266) directed against the central domain of Aβ could modify this equilibrium. Peripheral administration of m266 to PDAPP mice bound and sequestered all plasma Aβ and resulted in a rapid, massive increase in plasma Aβ as well as a reduction in Aβ deposition in the brain in chronically treated animals. Since amyloid plaques appear to abrogate the correlation between CNS and plasma Aβ, we assessed whether CNS to plasma Aβ efflux, as influenced by peripheral injection of m266, was indicative of brain amyloid load. Following intravenous administration of m266, we observed a rapid increase in plasma Aβ, and the magnitude of this increase was highly correlated with amyloid burden in the hippocampus and cortex of PDAPP mice. Together, these results suggest that there is a dynamic equilibrium between CNS and plasma Aβ and that certain anti-Aβ antibodies can act as a "peripheral sink" and alter this equilibrium.

Introduction

Amyloid-β (Aβ) is a normally soluble 39-43 amino peptide produced at highest levels in the CNS. Genetic and biochemical data strongly suggest that the conversion of Aβ from soluble to insoluble forms with high β-sheet content and its

---

[1] From the Center for the Study of Nervous System Injury
[2] Alzheimer's Disease Research Center
[3] Dept. of Neurology
[4] Molecular Biology and Pharmacology
[5] Washington University School of Medicine, 660 S. Euclid Ave., Box 8111, St. Louis, MO 63110; Neuroscience Discovery Research, Lilly Research Laboratories, Indianapolis, IN 46285

Selkoe/Christen
Immunization Against Alzheimer's Disease
and Other Neurodegenerative Disorders
© Springer-Verlag Berlin Heidelberg 2003

buildup in the brain is a key step in the pathogenesis of Alzheimer's disease (AD) and cerebral amyloid angiopathy (CAA; Golde et al. 2000). Prevention and/or reversal of this process may serve as a treatment. Methods to prevent or reverse Aβ deposition and its toxic effects would include decreasing its production, preventing its conversion to insoluble forms (e.g., inhibit β-sheet formation) or changing the dynamics of extracellular brain Aβ, either locally within the brain or by altering net flux of Aβ between the central nervous system (CNS) and plasma compartment. Transgenic mouse models of AD that develop age-dependent Aβ deposition, damage to the neuropil, and behavioral deficits have enabled researchers to test whether different manipulations can influence these AD-like changes (Price et al. 1998; Sisodia 1999). Recently, active immunization with different forms of the Aβ peptide has been shown to decrease brain Aβ deposition and improve cognitive performance in mouse models of AD (Schenk et al. 1999; Janus et al. 2000; Morgan et al. 2000, 2001; Weiner et al. 2000; Sigurdsson et al. 2001). Certain peripherally administered anti-Aβ antibodies have similar effects (Bard et al. 2000; DeMattos et al. 2001). The mechanism(s) by which anti-Aβ antibodies result in these effects is just beginning to be elucidated.

It has been speculated that one mechanism by which peripherally administered anti-Aβ antibodies influence Aβ deposition and possibly cognitive function is by crossing the blood-brain-barrier and subsequently 1) binding to plaques to mediate local clearance via microglia, 2) binding to aggregated Aβ to cause direct dissolution or 3) binding to toxic-soluble species of Aβ in the brain to block their effects. We have explored an alternative mechanism, in which certain anti-Aβ antibodies sequester plasma Aβ and act as a "peripheral sink" to facilitate increased efflux and clearance of Aβ from the CNS to the periphery. Herein, we present evidence supporting this mechanism.

Results

Human CNS and Plasma Aβ Appear to Be in Equilibrium in PDAPP Mice

Studies in animals suggest that exogenously administered ^{125}I-labeled Aβ can be transported bi-directionally from plasma to CNS and from CNS to plasma (Zlokovic et al. 1994, 1996; Poduslo et al. 1999; Shibata et al. 2000; DeMattos et al. 2001; Ji et al. 2001). We wanted to investigate whether mechanisms may also exist to modulate the transport of endogenously produced soluble pools of human Aβ between the CNS and plasma compartments. To begin to answer this question, we quantitated the level of Aβ in plasma and CSF of PDAPP mice as described (DeMattos et al. 2001; 2002b). PDAPP transgenic mice serve as a model in which a human APP transgene with a familial AD mutation is expressed almost exclusively in the brain (DeMattos et al. 2001) and which develop age-dependent Aβ/amyloid deposition (Games et al. 1995). To assess CSF Aβ levels, we developed a technique to reproducibly obtain 15-30 μl of non-plasma contaminated murine CSF (DeMattos et al. 2002b). The keys to the technique are isolating the CSF from the cisterna magna, utilizing anesthetized but live mice, and performing the isolation with the mouse in an inverted position with the aid of a dissecting microscope. In assessing human Aβ levels from CSF and plasma of young (three-month-old) PDAPP mice, prior to the appearance of Aβ deposition in the brain, we found that there was a highly significant positive correlation between the concentration of $Aβ_{Total}$ in CSF and plasma (r^2 = 0.6392, p = <0.0001, Fig. 1A). Since human APP in PDAPP mice is present almost exclusively in the CNS (DeMattos et al. 2001), this finding suggests that endogenously produced, soluble Aβ in the CNS is in equilibrium with Aβ in plasma. To investigate whether the development of Aβ deposition in the brain influenced the relationship between soluble Aβ in the CNS and plasma, we assessed CSF and plasma Aβ in nine-month-old PDAPP mice, an age at which some but not all mice had developed Aβ deposition in plaques. As was seen with three-month-old mice, there was a significant positive correlation between the concentration of $Aβ_{Total}$ in CSF and plasma in nine-month-old PDAPP mice (r^2 = 0.2532, p = 0.0170; Fig. 1B). Because the correlation

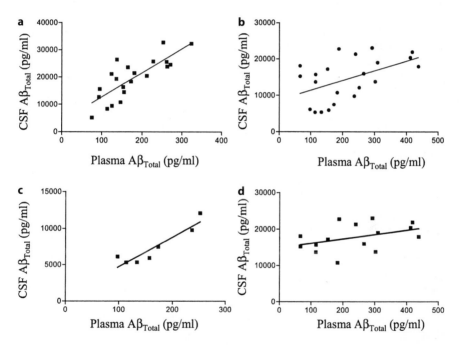

Fig. 1. Correlations between Aβ in CSF and plasma in PDAPP mice: modulation by plaques. Plasma and CSF were isolated from three- and nine-month-old PDAPP transgenic mice. $Aβ_{Total}$ levels were determined by radioimmunoassay (RIA). (A) A robust significant positive correlation was identified between the concentration of $Aβ_{Total}$ in CSF and plasma (r^2 = 0.6392, p < 0.0001) in three-month-old mice. (B) A weaker positive correlation was detected between CSF and plasma in nine-month-old mice (r^2 = 0.2532, p = 0.0170). (C) A significant positive correlation was identified between the concentration of $Aβ_{Total}$ in CSF and plasma (r^2 = 0.8572, p = 0.0028) in non-plaque- bearing nine-month-old mice. (D) No correlation was detected between CSF and plasma in plaque-bearing nine-month-old mice (r^2 = 0.1711, p = 0.1253). Reproduced with permission from DeMattos et al. (2002).

was much stronger in young vs. old PDAPP mice, we investigated whether the presence or absence of plaques modified the correlation in nine-month-old mice. When PDAPP mice with no Aβ deposition (no plaques) were analyzed separately, we detected a very robust correlation between $Aβ_{Total}$ in CSF and plasma ($r^2 = 0.8572$, p = 0.0028; Fig. 1C). In contrast, in plaque-bearing mice, there was no significant correlation between $Aβ_{Total}$ in CSF and plasma ($r^2 = 0.1711$, p = 0.1253; Fig. 1D). Together, these findings provide strong in vivo evidence that endogenous CNS and plasma Aβ are in a dynamic equilibrium and that the presence of plaques modifies this equilibrium.

Peripheral Anti-Aβ Antibody Alters CNS and Plasma Aβ Clearance and Decreases Brain Aβ Burden in a Mouse Model of AD

Previously, we reported that an anti-Aβ antibody (m266) present in the plasma could sequester plasma Aβ, alter the equilibrium between CNS and plasma Aβ and ultimately increase Aβ clearance from the CNS (DeMattos et al. 2001). We found that the baseline plasma concentration of human Aβ in PDAPP mice was ~150 pg/ml. We utilized a mouse monoclonal antibody directed against the central domain, residues 12-28 of Aβ (m266; Seubert et al. 1992), which was administered intravenously (i.v.) into three-month-old PDAPP mice. Twenty-four hours later, the concentration of free plasma Aβ not bound to antibody was undetectable (DeMattos et al. 2001). In contrast, the amount of plasma Aβ bound to m266 increased rapidly and markedly over time such that, by 24 to 72 hours following an i.v. dose of 600 μg, the Aβ concentration was ~100 ng/ml (~1000X higher than at baseline; Fig. 2). Further experiments in which exogenous Aβ was injected into the CSF space of wild-type mice in which m266 was present in the plasma also showed that a large fraction of Aβ injected in the CSF appeared in the plasma within minutes to hours (DeMattos et al. 2001). Lemere and colleagues (2001) recently reported that active immunization of another mouse model of AD (PSAPP) results in an increase in plasma Aβ. Since m266 had dramatic and rapid effects on plasma Aβ, we wanted to determine whether this antibody could also decrease Aβ deposition if given to PDAPP mice chronically. Thus, in a longer-term experiment, PDAPP[+/+] (homozygous) mice were treated with 500 μg of m266 every two weeks from four to nine months of age. Mice treated with m266 had significantly lower Aβ load (plaques) and Aβ levels in brain as compared to a saline and a control antibody-treated group (DeMattos et al. 2001).

These findings led us to hypothesize that certain circulating anti-Aβ antibodies, without crossing the blood-brain-barrier, may be able to alter the equilibrium between CNS and plasma Aβ, resulting in a net increase in Aβ efflux from the CNS. Several findings from this study suggest that the effects of circulating m266 resulting in a change in Aβ equilibrium contribute to both the rapid and chronic effects observed (Lee 2001). In regard to the rapid effects, a portion of the increase in plasma Aβ is likely due to m266 decreasing the normal degradation and clearance of plasma Aβ. However, effects of m266 on plasma Aβ levels in both wild-type and PDAPP mice along with acute effects on CSF Aβ, which could not

Fig. 2. Intravenous m266 detects rapid efflux of endogenous Aβ from CNS into plasma. In **(A)** and **(B)**, either 200 μg (n = 3) or 600 μg (n = 3) of m266 was injected i.v. into three-month-old APP^V717F +/+ mice. Prior to and at different time points following i.v. injection, the plasma concentration of Aβ bound to m266 was determined by radioimmunoassay. Each value is presented as mean +/- SEM. In **(A)**, the amount of Aβ bound to m266 is illustrated up to four days after treatment; in **(B)** the time course over the first several hours for all animals is shown. Reproduced with permission from DeMattos et al. (2001).

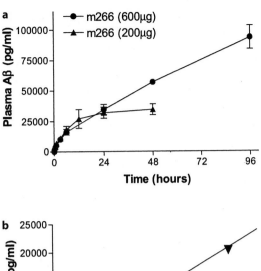

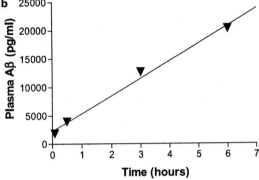

be accounted for by the very small amount of m266 measured in the CSF, suggest that m266 is altering the Aβ equilibrium between compartments. For example 24 hours following the i.v. injection of 500 μg of m266, the CSF concentration of $Aβ_{40}$ increased from 10 to 30 ng/ml (DeMattos et al. 2001). We directly assessed the concentration of m266 in the CSF 24 hours following i.v. administration and found it to be 12 ng/ml. If all of this antibody in the CSF was bound to Aβ, it would only result in an increase in the Aβ concentration by ~ 1 ng/ml. Thus, direct entry of the anti-Aβ antibody appears unlikely to have accounted for most of the acute effects on CSF Aβ that we observed. In regard to the chronic, plaque-lowering effects of m266, we found no evidence that m266 was bound to Aβ in plaques, despite the fact that, when directly applied to brain sections, this antibody did stain plaques. Finally, in recent experiments, we have found that peripherally administered m266 has rapid effects on cognition in older PDAPP mice at time points at which plaque-lowering effects are not yet observed (Dodart et al. 2001). Such effects may be due to circulating m266 rapidly altering the concentration of a soluble form of Aβ through alterations in a CNS/plasma Aβ equilibrium.

CNS to Plasma Amyloid-β Efflux: A Quantitative Measure of Brain Amyloid Burden in PDAPP Mice

Our studies indicated that human Aβ in CNS and plasma of PDAPP mice appeared to be in an equilibrium and that the equilibrium was modified by both insoluble forms of Aβ in the CNS (e.g., plaques) and the presence of an anti-Aβ antibody in the plasma (DeMattos et al. 2001, 2002b). Further, once PDAPP mice develop plaques, we found there was no longer a correlation between CSF and plasma Aβ or a correlation between Aβ load in brain (plaque load) and plasma Aβ (DeMattos et al. 2002b). We reasoned that plaques might alter the efflux rate of Aβ from the CNS to the blood and that the administration of an anti-Aβ antibody such as m266 would influence the efflux of Aβ from the CNS in a plaque-dependent manner. If this was the case and there was a relationship between plaque or Aβ load and the accumulation of Aβ in plasma in the presence of m266, then the administration of m266 followed by assessment of plasma Aβ would reflect or correlate with Aβ load. To test this idea, we assessed baseline levels of plasma Aβ from a cohort of 49 12- to 13-month-old PDAPP$^{+/+}$ mice. We then injected 500 μg of m266 i.v. and assessed plasma levels at various time points up to 24 hours later. Mice were then sacrificed and levels of plasma Aβ were compared to Aβ and amyloid load in the hippocampus and cortex. Importantly, while all PDAPP$^{+/+}$ mice ultimately develop Aβ deposits in the form of diffuse and neuritic (thioflavine-S-positive, amyloid) plaques after six months, there is a rather large variability in the degree of amyloid pathology in individual animals of the same age (DeMattos et al. 2001, 2002a; Fishman et al. 2001). This inherent variability in amyloid burden in our age-matched cohort allowed us to determine if plasma Aβ levels before or after m266 administration correlated with brain Aβ burden. In each plasma sample, levels of Aβ$_{40}$ and Aβ$_{42}$ were assessed by ELISA as previously described (DeMattos et al. 2001). Mice were sacrificed after 24 hours. One hemisphere was assessed using quantitative Aβ-immunofluorescent and thioflavine-S (amyloid) staining to determine the area of the hippocampus or cingulate cortex occupied by Aβ and amyloid, respectively (% Aβ or amyloid load), and regions from the other hemisphere were assessed for Aβ by ELISA as described (Holtzman et al. 2000; DeMattos et al. 2001; Fishman et al. 2001). Neuropathological assessment of Aβ and amyloid load was carried out by investigators blind to the plasma Aβ levels.

Fig. 3. Plasma levels of Aβ$_{40}$ following m266 administration are highly correlated with amyloid burden in hippocampus. Just before and following the i.v. administration of m266 (500 μg), plasma samples were collected at various times (e.g., 5 minutes and 24 hr). Plasma Aβ$_{40}$ was measured by ELISA and the percentage of the hippocampus covered by thioflavine-S positive material (% Amyloid deposition) was quantitated after sacrificing the mice. Prior to m266 administration, there was no correlation between the plasma levels of Aβ$_{40}$ and percentage of amyloid deposition in the hippocampus. In contrast, at 5 minutes and 24 hours following i.v. administration of m266, there were highly significant correlations (Pearson r values) when comparing the plasma levels of Aβ$_{40}$ to amyloid load in the hippocampus. Reproduced with permission from DeMattos et al. (2002).

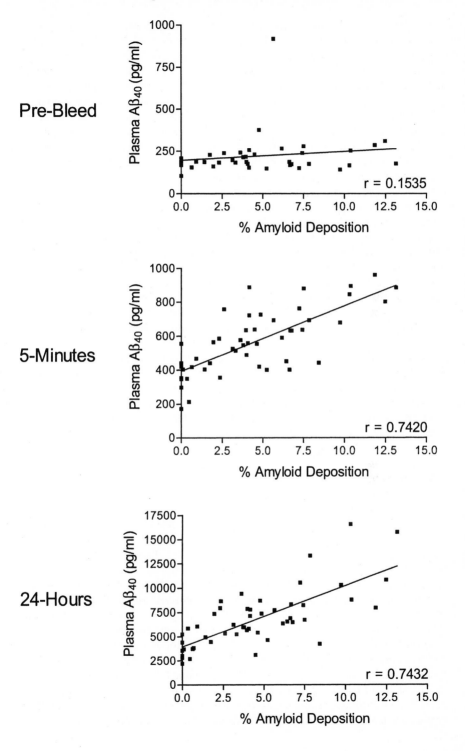

Baseline levels of plasma $A\beta_{40}$ (Fig. 3), $A\beta_{42}$, and the calculated $A\beta_{40/42}$ ratio prior to the administration of m266 did not correlate with the amount of $A\beta$ or amyloid deposition present in the brain (DeMattos et al. 2002a). This finding is similar to results seen in humans, where plasma $A\beta$ has been shown not to be a useful biomarker in distinguishing AD patients from age-matched controls (Mehta et al. 2000). As we have previously reported, following parenteral (i.v.) administration of m266, there was a rapid and marked increase in plasma $A\beta_{40}$ and $A\beta_{42}$. Importantly, following m266 administration, we observed highly significant correlations between levels of plasma $A\beta$ ($A\beta_{40}$) and both $A\beta$ and amyloid burden in the hippocampus (Fig. 3) and the cingulate cortex. Significant correlations were seen as early as five minutes following i.v. administration of m266 (Fig. 3). We also observed highly significant correlations when comparing $A\beta_{42}$, the $A\beta_{40/42}$ ratio and the total amount of plasma $A\beta_{40}$ and $A\beta_{42}$ accumulated over 24 hours (area under the curve, AUC) and both $A\beta$ and amyloid burden (DeMattos et al. 2002a). We next grouped mice according to their $A\beta$ burden and compared plasma $A\beta$ levels between those with the lowest, middle two, and highest quartiles of $A\beta$ burden. Significantly, there was no overlap in plasma $A\beta_{40}$ levels assessed at 24 hours (or in AUC for plasma $A\beta_{40}$) following m266 administration between mice in the lowest quartile (0–1.4%) vs. those in the highest quartile (18.2–34.5%) of brain $A\beta$ load (DeMattos et al. 2002a). By contrast, plasma $A\beta$ levels measured just prior to m266 administration failed to differentiate these two groups of mice (DeMattos et al. 2002a).

The findings of highly significant correlations between plasma $A\beta$ and both brain $A\beta$ and amyloid burden strongly suggest that the presence of m266 in the peripheral circulation directly facilitated net $A\beta$ efflux from the brain, acting as a "peripheral sink." By increasing $A\beta$ efflux from brain, it appears that the presence of m266 in plasma can also reveal quantitative differences in brain $A\beta$ deposition, presumably by facilitating efflux of soluble $A\beta$ from brain.

Discussion

There is now a relatively clear understanding of the cell biology underlying the production of $A\beta$ from APP and the molecules involved in the regulation of this process. Much less is known about $A\beta$ metabolism once it is released into the extracellular space either within or outside of the CNS. Recent evidence now suggests that the bi-directional transport of $A\beta$ between the CNS and plasma may play an important role in regulating brain $A\beta$ levels (Shibata et al. 2000). Studies have shown that exogenous $A\beta_{40}$ is rapidly transported from CSF to plasma, with an elimination half-life of ≤ 30 minutes (Ghersi-Egea et al. 1996; Shibata et al. 2000). In addition, there appear to be efficient receptor-mediated transport mechanisms for $A\beta$ at the blood-brain-barrier (Zlokovic et al. 1993, 1994, 1996 Poduslo et al. 1999; Shibata et al. 2000; Ji et al. 2001) that can be bi-directional; $A\beta$ is transported from CNS to plasma and from plasma to CNS. Our finding that levels of CSF and plasma $A\beta$ strongly correlate in young PDAPP mice and in older PDAPP mice without plaques suggests that endogenously produced human $A\beta$ in vivo also is transported across the blood-brain barrier and that CNS and plasma

Aβ pools are in equilibrium. Our finding that CSF and plasma Aβ levels do not correlate in PDAPP mice with plaques suggests that aggregated Aβ in vivo is altering the equilibrium of soluble CNS and plasma Aβ. This may be in some way be related to the fact that aggregated Aβ in vitro and in brain slices influences the local equilibrium between soluble and aggregated forms (Maggio et al. 1992; Esler et al. 2000). While changes in soluble Aβ binding molecules in the CNS (such as aggregated Aβ or apolipoprotein E) may alter CNS/plasma Aβ equilibrium, data following the peripheral injection of m266 in PDAPP mice also suggest that certain anti-Aβ antibodies such as m266 can also alter CNS/plasma Aβ equilibrium. The fact that peripheral injection of m266 results in 1) rapid and marked changes in plasma Aβ, 2) rapid changes in CSF Aβ, 3) a decrease in Aβ burden after chronic administration and rapid changes in cognition without staining plaques in the brain, and 4) accumulation of plasma Aβ, which is directly related to Aβ and amyloid load, all suggest a novel mechanism for altering CNS Aβ (DeMattos et al. 2001, 2002a). It is likely that m266 is either increasing efflux of Aβ from CNS to plasma and/or decreasing Aβ influx from plasma into CNS (DeMattos et al. 2001). Our understanding of the detailed mechanism(s) of Aβ transport across the blood-brain barrier is likely to be facilitated by studies utilizing anti-Aβ antibodies. Taken together, our data suggest that brain Aβ clearance is a dynamic process and that modifying this process may be useful in both diagnosing and treating AD.

Acknowledgments

This work was supported by Eli-Lilly, Inc. DMH was also supported by NIH grant AG20222.

References

Bard F, Cannon C, Barbour R, Burke R-L, Games D, Grajeda H, Guido T, Hu K, Huang J, Johnson-Wood K, Khan K, Kholodenko D, Lee M, Lieberburg I, Motter R, Nguyen M, Soriano F, Vasquez N, Weiss K, Welch B, Seubert P, Schenk D, TY (2000) Peripherally administered antibodies against amyloid β-peptide enter the central nervous system and reduce pathology in a mouse model of Alzheimer's disease. Nature Med 6:916–919

DeMattos RB, Bales KR, Cummins DJ, Dodart J-C, Paul SM, Holtzman DM (2001) Peripheral anti-Aβ antibody alters CNS and plasma Aβ clearance and decreases brain Aβ burden in a mouse model of Alzheimer's disease. Proc Natl Acad Sci USA 98:8850–8855

DeMattos RB, Bales KR, Cummins DJ, Paul SM, Holtzman DM (2002a) Brain to plasma amyloid-β efflux: A measure of brain amyloid burden in a mouse model of Alzheimer's disease. Science, 295:2264–2267

DeMattos RB, Bales KR, Parsadanian M, Kierson ME, O'Dell MA, Foss EM, Paul SM, Holtzman DM (2002b) Plaque-associated disruption of CSF and plasma Ab equilibrium in a mouse model of Alzheimer's Disease. J Neurochem, 81:229–236

Dodart J-C, Bales KR, DeMattos RB, Mathis C, Delong CA, Wu X, Holtzman DM, Paul SM (2001) Passive immunization reverses memory deficits but not Alzheimer-like pathology in very old APPV717F transgenic mice. Soc Neurosci Abstr 27:687.12

Esler WP, Stimson ER, Jennings JM, Vinters HV, Ghilardi JR, Lee JP, Mantyh PW, Maggio JE (2000) Alzheimer's disease amyloid propagation by a template-dependent dock-lock mechanism. Biochemistry 39:6288–6295

Fishman CE, Cummins DJ, Bales KR, DeLong CA, Esterman MA, Hanson JC, L. WS, Paul SM, Jordan WH (2001) Statistical aspects of quantitative image analysis of beta-amyloid in the APP(V717F) transgenic mouse model of Alzheimer's disease. J Neurosci Meth 108:145–152

Games D, Adams D, Alessandrini R, Barbour R, Berthelette P, Blackwell C, Carr T, Clemens J, Donaldson T, Gillespie F, Guido T, Hagopian S, Johnson-Wood K, Khan K, Lee M, Leibowitz P, Lieberburg I, Little S, Masliah E, McConlogue L, Montoya-Zavala, Mucke L, Paganini L, Penniman E, Power M, Schenk D, Seubert P, Snyder B, Soriano F, Tan H, Vitale J, Wadsworth S, Wolozin B, Zhao J (1995) Alzheimer-type neuropathology in transgenic mice overexpressing V717F β-amyloid precursor protein. Nature 373:523–527

Ghersi-Egea J-F, Gorevic PD, Ghiso J, Frangione B, Patlak CS, Fensternacher JD (1996) Fate of cerebrospinal fluid-borne amyloid [beta]-peptide: Rapid clearance into blood and appreciable accumulation by cerebral arteries. J Neurochem 67:880–883

Golde TE, Eckman CB, Younkin SG (2000) Biochemical detection of Aβ isoforms: implications for pathogenesis, diagnosis, and treatment of Alzheimer's disease. Biochim Biophys Acta 1502:172–187

Holtzman DM, Bales KR, Tenkova T, Fagan AM, Parsadanian M, Sartorius LJ, Mackey B, Olney J, McKeel D, Wozniak D, Paul SM (2000) Apolipoprotein E isoform-dependent amyloid deposition and neuritic degeneration in a mouse model of Alzheimer's disease. Proc Natl Acad Sci USA 97:2892–2897

Janus C, Pearson J, McLaurin J, Mathews PM, Jiang Y, Schmidt SD, Chishti MA, Horne P, Heslin D, French J, Mount HTJ, Nixon RA, Mercken M, Bergeron C, Fraser PE, St. George-Hyslop P, Westaway D (2000) Aβ peptide immunization reduced behavioural impairment and plaques in a model of Alzheimer' s disease. Nature 408:979–982

Ji Y, Permanne B, Sigurdsson EM, Holtzman DM, Wisniewski T (2001) Amyloid β40/42 clearance across the blood-brain barrier following intraventricular injections in wild-type, apoE knock-out and human apoE3 or E4 expressing transgenic mice. J Alzheimer's Dis 3:23–30

Lee VM-Y (2001) Aβ immunization: Moving Aβ peptide from brain to blood. Proc Natl Acad Sci USA 98:8931–8932

Lemere CA, Spooner ET, Malester B, LaFrancois J, C.Mori C, Leverone JF, Clements JT, Selkoe DJ, Duff KE (2001) Aβ immunization of PSAPP mice leads to decreased cerebral Aβ and a corresponding increase in serum Aβ. Soc Neurosci Abstr 27:687.10

Maggio J, Stimson E, Ghilardi J, Allen C, Dahl C, Whitcomb D, Vigna S, Vinters H, Labenski M, Mantyh P (1992) Reversible in vitro growth of Alzheimer disease beta-amyloid plaques by deposition of labeled amyloid peptide. Proc Natl Acad Sci USA 89:5462–5466

Mehta PD, Pirttila T, Mehta SP, Sersen EA, Aisen PS, Wisniewski HM (2000) Plasma and cerebrospinal fluid levels of amyloid β proteins 1-40 and 1-42 in Alzheimer's disease. Arch Neurol 57:100–105

Morgan D, Diamond DM, Gottschall PE, Ugen KE, Dickey C, Hardy J, Duff K, Jantzen P, Dicarlo G, Wilcock D, Connor K, Hatcher J, Hope C, Gordon M, Arendash GW (2000) Aβ peptide vaccination prevents memory loss in an animal model of Alzheimer's disease. Nature 408:982–985

Morgan D, Diamond DM, Gottschall PE, Ugen KE, Dickey C, Hardy J, Duff K, Jantzen P, Dicarlo G, Wilcock D, Connor K, Hatcher J, Hope C, Gordon M, Arendash GW (2001) Aβ peptide vaccination prevents memory loss in an animal model of Alzheimer's disease (Correction). Nature 412:660

Poduslo JF, Curran GL, Sanyal B, Selkoe DJ (1999) Receptor-mediated transport of human amyloid beta-protein 1-40 and 1-42 at the blood-brain barrier. Neurobiol Dis 6:190–199

Price DL, Sisodia SS, Borchelt DR (1998) Genetic neurodegenerative diseases: the human illness and transgenic models. Science 282:1079–1083

Schenk D, Barbour R, Dunn W, Gordon G, Grajeda H, Guido T, Hu K, Huang J, Johnson-Wood K, Khan K, Kholodenko D, Lee M, Liao Z, Lieberburg I, Motter R, Mutter L, Soriano F, Shopp G,

Vasquez N, Vandevert C, Walker S, Wogulis M, Yednock T, Games D, Seubert P (1999) Immunization with amyloid-beta attenuates Alzheimer-disease-like pathology in the PDAPP mouse. Nature 400:173–177

Seubert P, Vigo-Pelfrey C, Esch F, Lee M, Dovey H, David D, Sinha S, Schlossmacher M, Whaley J, Swindlehurst C, McCormack R, Wolfert R, Selkoe D, Lieberburg I, Schenk D (1992) Isolation and quantification of soluble Alzheimer's β-peptide from biological fluids. Nature 359:325–327

Shibata M, Yamada S, Kumar SR, Calero M, Bading J, Frangione B, Holtzman DM, Miller CA, Strickland DK, Ghiso J, Zlokovic BV (2000) Clearance of Alzheimer's amyloid-β1-40 peptide from brain by LDL receptor–related protein-1 at the blood-brain barrier. J Clin Invest 106:1489–1499

Sigurdsson EM, Scholtzova H, Mehta P, Frangione B, Wisniewski T (2001) Immunization with a nontoxic/nonfibrillar amyloid-β homologous peptide reduces Alzheimer's disease-associated pathology in transgenic mice. Am J Pathol 159:439–447

Sisodia SS (1999) Alzheimer's disease: perspectives for the new millennium. J Clin Invest 104:1169–1170

Weiner HL, Lemere CA, Maron R, Spooner ET, Grenfell TJ, Mori C, Issazadeh S, Hancock WW, Selkoe DJ (2000) Nasal administration of amyloid-β peptide decreases cerebral amyloid burden in a mouse model of Alzheimer's disease. Ann Neurol 48:567–579

Zlokovic BV, Ghiso J, Mackic JB, McComb JG, Weiss MH, Frangione B (1993) Blood-brain barrier transport of circulating Alzheimer's amyloid β. Biochem Biophys Res Comm 197:1034–1040

Zlokovic BV, Martel CL, Mackic JB, Matsubara E, Wisniewski T, McComb JG, Frangione B, Ghiso J (1994) Brain uptake of circulating apolipoproteins J and E complexed to Alzheimer's amyloid β. Biochem Biophys Res Commun 205:1431–1437

Zlokovic BV, Martel CL, Matsubara E, McComb JG, Zheng G, McCluskey RT, Frangione B, Ghiso J (1996) Glycoprotein 330/megalin: probable role in receptor-mediated transport of apolipoprotein J alone and in a complex with Alzheimer's disease amyloid β at the blood-brain and blood-cerebrospinal fluid barriers. Proc Natl Acad Sci USA 93:4229–4234

Multiphoton Microscopy: Imaging Plaques and Reversal of Plaques – a Transgenic Model by Multiphoton Microscopy

B.T. Hyman and B. J. Bacskai

The Problem: Aβ Deposition Occurs Throughout the Brain, Forming Large Aggregates: Are These Reversible?

Early-onset, autosomal-dominant Alzheimer's disease patients share their mutations in the gene for amyloid precursor protein (APP) or in the presenilin gene, thought to be important in APP processing to Aβ, leading to a phenotype of elevated Aβ deposition in the brain and early onset dementia (see Selkoe 2000 for review).

These data place Aβ deposition central to Alzheimer pathophysiology and support the idea that amyloid deposition initiates a cascade of events ultimately leading to neuronal loss and dementia.

In formulating therapies for Alzheimer's disease, a central paradox exists: if Aβ deposits that occur in the brain are large, stable aggregates, then reducing Aβ generation may not be sufficient to reduce plaques that have already formed. Since amyloid plaques are abundant throughout cortical and limbic areas in the brains of patients who have just the very beginning of symptoms of dementia due to Alzheimer's disease, the therapeutic challenge is great: if these plaques cannot be reversed, the best one might hope for is stabilization of the process. On the other hand, if the Aβ deposits are reversible, the hope would remain that, at least to some extent, the neuronal alterations associated with plaques might also be remediable.

The natural history of plaques is essentially unknown. Because they are difficult to solubilize biochemically, requiring harsh conditions such as formic acid extraction, they are generally thought to be stable and long-lived. Some biochemical evidence supports this point of view, suggesting extensive cross-linking within densely fibrillar plaques. On the other hand, a detailed analysis of Aβ deposit microstructure showed that the size distribution of plaques was log normal, consistent with the physical structure obtained by amphipathic substances in equilibrium with an aqueous environment (Hyman et al. 1995; Cruz et al. 1997). The exact size distribution and geometric features of Aβ deposits in the cortex were modeled by computer as a process that includes deposition of Aβ and then

Massachusetts General Hospital/Harvard Medical School, Department of Neurology, 114 16th Street (CAGN 2009), Charlestown, MA 02129, U.S.A.
Tel: (617)726-2299, (617)724-8330, Fax: (617)724-1480, E-Mail: B_Hyman@helix.mgh.harvard.edu, Bacskai@helix.mgh.harvard.edu

Selkoe/Christen
Immunization Against Alzheimer's Disease
and Other Neurodegenerative Disorders
© Springer-Verlag Berlin Heidelberg 2003

growth to a steady state; then feedback processes preclude further growth (Urbanc et al. 1999).

We have postulated that the activated microglia and astrocytes surrounding plaques might contribute to this stabilization of plaque size. However, since plaques are so small, they cannot be imaged in vivo with routine imaging devices such as SPECT or MRI. A new approach was needed to tackle the problem of whether or not plaques continue to grow, shrink, or are stable over time (i.e., the natural history of plaques) and whether treatment might allow them to be reversed. What emerges from our studies is the idea that Aβ deposition is a dynamic process, with rapid deposition and relatively slower feedback phenomena that ultimately lead to a steady state of amyloid deposits. Moreover, various morphological subtypes of plaques seem to affect the neuropil differentially, with dense core, Thioflavin-S positive plaques representing lesions that disrupt dendrites. Taken together, these results lead to a formulation of amyloid hypotheses that focus on focal, but distributed lesions scattered throughout the cortex. If this is the case, removal of plaques may prove to be helpful for restoration of neural system integrity.

Application of Multiphoton Microscopy to Imaging Plaques

In the last several years we have taken a radical new approach to develop methods to perform in vivo microscopy so that the pathophysiological processes can be directly observed over time. We have approached this goal by adapting a technique called multiphoton microscopy, which is similar in many ways to the more commonly used confocal microscope. In collaboration with Dr. Watt Webb, a physicist at Cornell University who invented multiphoton microscopy (Denk et al. 1990), we have developed an instrument for in vivo imaging of the cerebral cortex in the living mouse. We can now image multiple fluorophores in an anesthetized mouse, allowing in vivo histology, in vivo immunofluorescence, and in vivo functional imaging, all with the resolution equal to, or better than, confocal microscopy.

First we provide a description of the principles behind this novel form of microscopy. The basic principle behind the invention of multiphoton microscopy relies on the quantum physics of fluorescence excitation. An electron is excited to a higher energy state after absorbing energy from a photon with a characteristic wavelength. When that electron decays back down to its ground state, it releases a photon with a slightly longer wavelength. This corresponds to the absorption and emission of wavelengths of a fluorescent molecule (Fig. 1). If a fluorophore interacts with two photons, each containing one half of the characteristic energy needed to excite the molecule, the electron can reach its excited state provided that the two "half energy" photons interact with the molecule essentially simultaneously. The critical point is to have sufficient flux of photons within a small volume so that the probability of two of them interacting with a single fluorophore simultaneously is high.

Dr. Webb solved this problem using a high-powered, femtosecond-pulsed laser focused through a microscope objective. At the heart of the focal point of the objective, photon flux is sufficient to induce two-photon excitation. Denk and Svo-

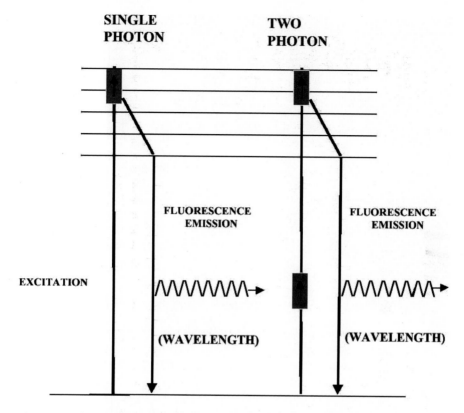

Fig. 1. Principle of multiphoton excitation, illustrating the energy states of electrons after fluorescent excitation by single or two-photon mechanisms.

boda illustrated this point by calculating that, for a molecule of rhodamine D exposed to sunlight, a single-photon excitation will occur once a second, but a two-photon event will spontaneously occur only once in 10 million years (Denk and Svoboda 1997).

For biological imaging, the advantages are substantial. We have noticed that wavelengths above 700 nm are less damaging to tissue than UV light. Secondly, longer wavelengths pass through translucent tissue to a greater depth. Standard confocal microscopes, for example, cannot penetrate much more than 40 microns from the surface of the tissue. Multiphoton microscopy allows penetration up to 400 microns. Thirdly, and of equal importance, is the way in which emitted light is collected. In standard microscopy, the entire thickness of the section is exposed to exciting light and consequently fluoresces. The deeper into the tissue one goes, the more scattering occurs. By contrast, in multiphoton microscopy, the only part of the tissue that can fluoresce is the very small volume at the exact heart of the focal plane of the objective lens. Thus, any light that is emitted, regardless of how much it is scattered, can be reassigned to that excitation volume. This has the ef-

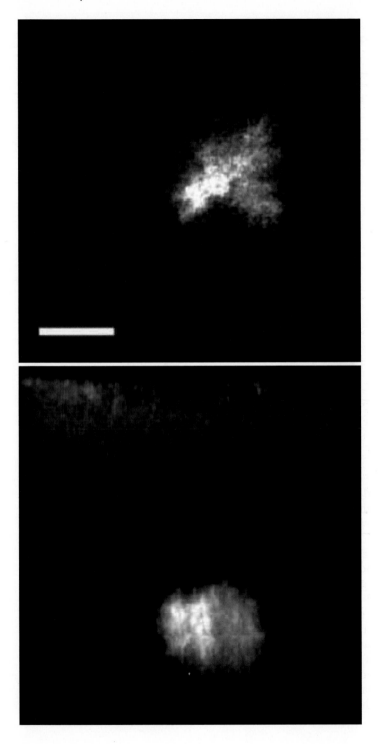

fect of improving resolution and signal-to-noise dramatically with the resolution in the XY plane of about 400 nm, as well as the beneficial biological effect of not exposing fluorophors above and below the optical plane of imaging to activating light. The small excitation volume is scanned over an XY field and the objective is moved in the Z axis in increments as small as 0.1 micron to develop a Z series stack of images which, when reconstructed, provide dramatic three-dimensional images.

In the last several years, the promise of this approach has been seen in a series of in vitro studies in cultured cells as slice preparations (see Denk and Svoboda 1997). Some important applications of the central nervous system have followed; for example, alterations of the shape of dendritic spines during induction of long-term potentiation have been visualized (Koester et al. 1999). Beautiful images of calcium flux (Denk et al. 1995) in neurons in response to sensory input have been obtained in rat cortex in acute surgical preparations (Svoboda et al. 1999).

We have developed this technique to image pathological features in living transgenic mice and can now image both Thioflavin-S positive (Fig. 2) and immunoreactive Aβ deposits in the living mouse. We have also developed additional reagents and approaches that allow us to monitor three channels of optical information simultaneously, giving us the potential to also record neuronal structure and function. We image a volume about 600 micrometers wide X 600 micrometers long X 200-300 micrometers deep to the surface. Although the mouse is anesthetized during the imaging, after imaging it recovers well and it can be re-imaged hours to days to months later.

Because the mouse sits on a stereotax on an XY encoded stage, and because we record a fluorescent angiogram at the same time of imaging, we are able to readily re-image exactly the same volume of cortex and match the reconstructed three-dimensional volumes to each other with outstanding accuracy (Christie et al. 2000).

Imaging of plaques in PDAPP mice and in Tg2576 mice lead to similar and surprising results. Imaging Thioflavin-S as the fluorescent marker for plaques, we found that plaques form rather quickly and then reach a stable size and shape that remains stable for months thereafter. We have imaged and re-imaged over 300 plaques in mice over time intervals ranging from days to five months (Christie et al. 2000). The plaque number and size appear to be stable over this time course, giving us a stable readout for reversal therapies.

Reversal of Plaques by Anti-Aβ Antibody Administration

Having achieved the ability to image plaques in vivo, we could then ask the question of whether or not they could be reversed. Schenk et al. (1999) showed elegantly that immunization with Aβ could prevent plaque formation in PDAPP mice. The implication was that Aβ monomers, or perhaps small aggregates, were being cleared before they could gather to precipitate into plaques. Further study

---

Fig. 2. In vivo imaging of a plaque stained by Thioflavine-S. The lower panel is a three-dimensional reconstruction of the plaque. Bar = 10 micrometers.

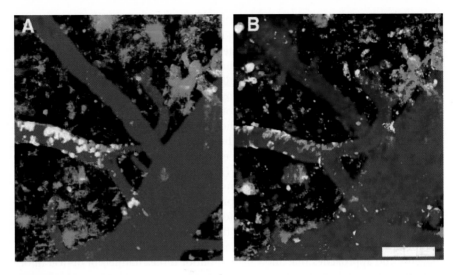

Fig. 3. In vivo multiphoton imaging of amyloid-β deposits visualized by 10D5 (a) and then, three days later, by BAM-10. Bar = 90 micrometers.

by Bard et al. (2000) showed clearly that passive immunization was sufficient for this purpose as well and could prevent amyloid deposits. These are extraordinarily exciting observations, but do not directly address the question that we were most interested in: can existing plaques be reversed?

To tackle this question, we used PDAPP mice and imaged plaques at baseline. We carried out this imaging in two ways: first, using Thioflavin-S as a histochemical marker of amyloid deposits and also using directly labeled anti-Aβ antibody (10d5). The fluorescently labeled antibody was applied directly to the cortical surface, and after 20 minutes the mouse was imaged. This procedure provided an in vivo immunofluorescent reporter for the presence of plaques and amyloid angiopathy that was quite robust (Fig. 3). Diffuse plaques, dense core plaques, and amyloid angiopathy were all easily visualized within 100 to 200 microns of the surface, the diffusion limit of the antibody.

We re-imaged the mice three to seven days later, using Thioflavin-S again, fluorescently labeled 10d5, or fluorescently labeled anti-amyloid antibodies that do not have a cross-reacting epitope with 10d5. While the exact numbers vary depending on which of these readouts we use, the striking result is that the vast majority of plaques that had been present at baseline are cleared by the antibody treatment (Bacskai et al. 2000). For example, about 70% of Thioflavin-S plaques initially visualized were cleared after antibody treatment, whereas in the control, only about 20% of the Thioflavin-S plaques could not be revisualized (P<0.001; (Bacskai et al. 2000).

We have screened a variety of anti-Aβ antibodies and have the impression that antibodies directed against the N terminal portion of Aβ are more effective at clearance. For example, 3d6, 10d5, and the commercially available BAM-10

(Sigma) all clear Aβ deposits with similar efficacy. By contrast, our preliminary studies with antibodies targeted to the mid or carboxy terminus of Aβ are less effective at both in vivo imaging and clearance.

Our most recent studies involve asking the question of whether Fc-mediated uptake of the antibodies is a critical element. Bard et al. (2000) showed that microglia can interact with plaques that have been decorated by antibodies via Fc-mediated mechanisms in an ex vivo preparation. While it seems likely to us that this occurs in vivo as well, several observations suggest that the picture is more complex. Solomon and colleagues (1997) suggested that Aβ antibodies might dissociate plaques via simple biophysical interaction by breaking up β-pleated sheet conformation. In accordance with this possibility, our preliminary data suggest that Fab-2 fragments of antibodies are also rather effective at clearing existing Aβ deposits. Aβ plaques shrink substantially over just three days. While still preliminary, these data suggest that non-Fc-mediated mechanisms may well be implicated in clearance of existing plaques by antibodies.

Future Directions

The advent of multiphoton microscopy for imaging of plaques opens up a wide variety of investigations regarding the effect of amyloid deposition in the brain. For example, we have studied the effect of amyloid deposits on blood vessel function, taking advantage of the concurrent fluorescent angiogram and amyloid imaging afforded by the multiphoton microscope (Kimchi et al. 2001). These experiments led to several intriguing conclusions. Vessel segments that contain Aβ are significantly wider than adjacent parts of the same vessels that do not contain Aβ. This finding suggests that amyloid angiopathy leads to dysfunction of the normal tone of the cerebral microvasculature. We have directly addressed this question by studying vessel response to either acetylcholine or a nitric oxide donor and have demonstrated directly that, in Tg2576 mice, vascular smooth muscle dysfunction occurs even before smooth muscle cell loss (Christie et al. 2000).

We have also seen that amyloid angiopathy tends to start at points relatively near branch points of vessels and then grows from these "seeds" (Kimchi et al. 2001). This brings to mind some of the changes that occur early in atherosclerosis. It remains to be seen whether amyloid angiopathy can be prevented or reversed by antibody treatment, but it seems likely that the robust physiologic effect of the amyloid on blood vessel responses translates to another mechanism for neuronal dysfunction.

What else can multiphoton microscopy provide? We have developed a series of new in vivo imaging techniques, including staining with Hoechst dye for nuclei (and monitoring nuclear morphology), back labeling with labeled dextrans to provide detailed imaging of dendritic and axonal structure, and even delivery of EGFP and EGFP-tagged proteins via gene transfer techniques. While still in the early stages, we have sufficient results to provide great enthusiasm for this novel technique. We believe that we will have the tools to study the natural history of plaques, the response of various cellular elements to plaques, and the functional consequences of plaques in their microenvironment. Immunotherapy or similar techniques designed to clear plaques from the cortex can be directly tested, and the functional consequences of clearing plaques can be evaluated.

Acknowledgments

Supported by a grant from the Alzheimer's Association, NIH AG08487, and the Walter's Family Foundation.

References

Bacskai B, Kajdasz S, Christie R, Carter C, Games D, Seubert P, Schenk D, Hyman B (2001) Imaging of amyloid β deposits in brains of living mice permits direct observation of clearance of plaques with immunotherapy. Nature Med 7:369–372

Bard F, Cannon C, Barbour R, Burke RL, Games D, Grajeda H, Guido T, Hu K, Huang J, Johnson-Wood K, Khan K, Kholodenko D, Lee M, Lieberburg I, Motter R, Nguyen M, Soriano F, Vasquez N, Weiss K, Welch B, Seubert P, Schenk D, Yednock T (2000) Peripherally administered antibodies against amyloid eta-peptide enter the central nervous system and reduce pathology in a mouse model of Alzheiemer disease. Nature Med 6:916–919

Christie R, Yamada M, Moskowitz M, Hyman BT(2000) Structural and functional disruption of vascular smooth muscle cells in a transgenic mouse model of amyloid angiopathy. Am J Pathol 158:1065–1071

Christie R, Bacskai B, Zipfel W, Willimas R, Kajdasz S, Webb W, Hyman BT (2001) Growth arrest of individual senile plaques in a model of Alzheimer's disease observed by *in vivo* multiphoton microscopy. J Neurosci 21:858–864

Cruz L, Urbanc B, Buldyrev SV, Christie R, Gomez-Isla T, Havlin S, McNamara M, Stanley HE, Hyman BT (1997) Aggregation and disaggregation of senile plaques in Alzheimer disease. Proc Natl Acad Sci (USA) 94:7612–7616

Denk W, Svoboda K (1997) Photon upmanship: Why multiphoton imaging is more than a gimmick. Neuron 18:351–357

Denk W, Strickler JH, Webb WW (1990) Two-photon laser scanning fluorescence microscopy. Science 248:73-76

Denk W, Sugimori M, Llinas R (1995) Two types of calcium response limited to single spines in cerebellar Purkinje cells. Proc Natl Acad Sci (USA) 92:8279–8282

Hyman BT, West HL, Rebeck GW, Lai F, Mann DM. (1995) Neuropathological changes in Down's syndrome hippocampal formation. Effect of age and apolipoprotein E genotype. Arch Neurol 52:373–378

Kimchi E, Kajdasz S, Bacskai B, Hyman B (2001) Analysis of cerebral amyloid angiopathy in a transgenic mouse model of Alzheimer's disease using *in vivo* multiphoton microscopy. J Neuropath Exp Neurol 60:274–279

Koester HJ, Baur D, Uhl R, Hell SW (1999) Ca2+ fluorescence imaging with pico- and femtosecond two-photon excitation: Signal and photodamage. Biophys 77:2226–2236

Selkoe DJ (2000) The origins of Alzheimer disease: A is for amyloid. (Editorial comment) JAMA 283:1615–1617

Schenk D, Barbour R, Dunn W, Gordon G, Grajeda H, Guido T, Hu K, Huang J, Johnson-Wood K, Khan K, Kholodenko D, Lee M, Liao Z, Lieberburg I, Motter R, Mutter L, Soriano F, Shopp G, Vasquez N, Vendevert C, Walker S, Wogulis M, Yednock T, Games D, Seubert P (1999) Immunization with amyloid-β attenuates Alzheimer-disease-like pathology in the PDAPP mouse. Nature 400:173–177

Solomon B, Koppel R, Frankel D, Hanan-Aharon E (1997) Disaggregation of Alzheimer beta-amyloid by site-directed mAβ. Proc Natl Acad Sci (USA) 94:4109–4112

Svoboda K, Helmchen F, Denk W, Tank DW (1999) Spread of dendritic excitation in layer 2/3 pyramidal neurons in rat barrel cortex *in vivo*. Nature Neurosci 2:65–73

Urbanc B, Cruz L, Buldyrev SV, Havlin S, Stanley HE, Hyman BT (1999) Dynamic feedback in an aggregation-disaggregation model. Phys Rev E 60:2120–2126

Antibodies as Therapeutic Agents for Prion Disease

D. Peretz[1], R. A. Williamson[2], K. Kaneko[1,3], D. R. Burton[2] and S. B. Prusiner[1,4]

Summary

Prions are infectious proteins that cause fatal neurodegenerative disorders in humans and animals. The emergence of variant Creutzfeldt-Jakob disease (vCJD) in humans, which seems to be caused by the consumption of prion-infected beef, has heightened the urgency for developing effective therapeutic agents. Prions reproduce by recruiting normal prion protein (PrP^C) and stimulating its conversion to the disease-causing isoform (PrP^{Sc}): $PrP^{Sc} + PrP^C \rightarrow PrP^{Sc}PrP^C \rightarrow PrP^{Sc} + PrP^{Sc}$. This mechanism suggests that compounds specifically binding either PrP isoform may interrupt prion production by inhibiting this misfolding process. We and other researchers have demonstrated that antibodies specific to PrP inhibit prion propagation in cultured, prion-infected mouse neuroblastoma (ScN2a) cells (Peretz et al. 2001; Enari et al. 2001). In experiments by other researchers, transgenic mice expressing the heavy chain of an anti-PrP antibody were protected against prions inoculated intraperitoneally (Heppner et al. 2001). When we consider the mechanism of prion production in neuronal cell cultures and the binding properties of efficient antibodies, the inhibitory effect is most readily explained by antibodies binding specifically to PrP^C molecules on the cell surface and thereby hampering their transition to PrP^{Sc}. Significantly, in cells treated with the most potent antibody, D18, prion replication is completely abolished and pre-existing PrP^{Sc} is rapidly cleared, suggesting that antibodies may cure established infection. These data support the use of antibodies in the prevention and treatment of prion diseases.

Introduction

Deposits of specific proteins can be found in a large group of neurodegenerative diseases (Kaytor and Warren 1999) . The protein aggregates are generally dense fibrillar structures containing a high percentage of β-sheet structures. These pro-

---

[1] Institute for Neurodegenerative Diseases and Departments of Neurology and of [4]Biochemistry and Biophysics, University of California, San Francisco, CA 94143.
[2] Department of Immunology and Molecular Biology, The Scripps Research Institute, La Jolla, CA 92037.
[3] Present address: National Institute of Neuroscience, Tokyo 187-8502, Japan.

Selkoe/Christen
Immunization Against Alzheimer's Disease
and Other Neurodegenerative Disorders
© Springer-Verlag Berlin Heidelberg 2003

tein aggregates can be found extracellularly and in different cellular compartments. These neurodegenerative diseases may be sporadic or inherited because of mutations in a chromosomal gene.

Prion diseases, or transmissible spongiform encephalopathies (TSE[s]), comprise a group of fatal neurodegenerative disorders afflicting humans and animals. All involve aberrant metabolism of the prion protein (PrP), a constituent of normal mammalian cells. Prions are defined as proteinaceous infectious particles that are devoid of nucleic acid and seem to be composed exclusively of a disease-causing isoform of PrP, designated PrP^{Sc}. The normal, cellular PrP, denoted PrP^{C}, is converted into PrP^{Sc} through a process whereby some of its structure is converted into β-sheet (Caughey et al. 1991a; Gasset et al. 1993; Pan et al. 1993; Safar et al. 1993; Pergami et al. 1996). This structural transition is accompanied by profound changes in the physicochemical properties of PrP. PrP^{C} is readily soluble in non-denaturing detergents and is digested rapidly by proteases. In contrast, PrP^{Sc} is insoluble in such detergents and is resistant to proteolysis, except for the N-terminal region comprised of ~67 residues (Prusiner et al. 1983, 1984; Basler et al. 1986). The protease-resistant fragment of PrP^{Sc} has a molecular mass of 27 to 30 kDa and conveys prion infectivity (Prusiner et al. 1983, 1984; Basler et al. 1986; McKinley et al. 1983). Protein denaturants abolish prion infectivity and protease resistance while increasing solubility and facilitating immunodetection of PrP^{Sc} (Kitamoto et al. 1987; Serban et al. 1990; Taraboulos et al. 1992a; Prusiner et al. 1993a; Oesch et al. 1994; Peretz et al. 1997). Thus, considerable evidence argues that prion diseases are disorders of protein conformation.

Prion diseases exist as inherited, sporadic and infectious disorders. From the perspective of inherited and sporadic neurodegenerative diseases, Alzheimer's and prion diseases could share similar pathogenic mechanisms (Cohen and Prusiner 1998). However, a fundamental difference arises from the transmissibility of prion diseases, which has not been demonstrated with other neurodegenerative diseases. Transmission of tissue from animals suffering from prion disease causes disease in the recipient host. Evidence suggests that, following passage of prions between animals, incoming PrP^{Sc} interacts directly with PrP^{C} of the host, which leads to the faithful conversion of PrP^{C} to PrP^{Sc} (Prusiner et al. 1990; Telling et al. 1996; Horiuchi et al. 1999). The efficiency of the infection between hosts of the same species relates to the amount of prions in the inoculum (titer), mode of entry, and frequency of exposure. However, interspecies transmission of prions depends also on the homology of the donor and host PrP genes and the conformation of incoming PrP^{Sc} (Scott et al. 1989; Peretz et al. 2002). Transmissions of prions from person to person by contaminated neurosurgical instruments, corneal transplants, cadaveric dura mater grafts, human pituitary-derived growth hormone, and ritualistic cannibalism have been documented (Will et al. 1999).

Inherited prion diseases include Gerstmann-Sträussler-Scheinker disease (GSS), familial Creutzfeldt-Jakob disease (fCJD) and fatal familial insomnia (FFI). Molecular genetic studies argue that these diseases are caused by mutations in the PrP gene (Prusiner 1998). To explain inherited prion diseases, it has been suggested that the wild-type PrP^{C} prefers a monomeric state whereas mutant PrP^{C} preferentially adopts the disease-causing multimeric state, PrP^{Sc} (Cohen and Prusiner 1998). Once mutated PrP^{Sc} is formed, it facilitates the conversion process by acting as a template to which PrP^C binds and eventually adopts the pathological conformation.

Sporadic cases of prion disease could arise by the following two scenarios (Cohen and Prusiner 1998). First, a somatic mutation in neuronal cells could give rise to a mutant PrP^C that prefers the PrP^{Sc} conformation. Initially, propagation of PrP^{Sc} would be limited to the cell in which the somatic mutation had occurred, then would spread gradually through neuronal tissue and finally to the brain. Alternatively, a rare, spontaneous conformational rearrangement of PrP^C could lead to the formation and accumulation of PrP^{Sc}.

Biogenesis of PrP^C

The biosynthesis of PrP^C is similar to that of other glycoproteins. As PrP polypeptide chains are elongated, the signal peptide of 22 amino acids at the NH_2-terminus is removed, as for other secretory proteins (Basler et al. 1986; Hope et al. 1986; Turk et al. 1988). After assembly of the polypeptide chain is complete, a signal sequence of 23 amino acids is removed from the COOH-terminus and a glycosylphosphatidylinositol (GPI) anchor is added at position 231 (Stahl et al. 1987, 1990). From the Golgi, PrP^C molecules continue to the cell surface where they are attached to the external surface of the plasma membrane by the GPI anchor (Stahl et al. 1987, 1992). PrP^C can be released from the cell surface upon treatment with phosphatidylinositol-specific phospholipase C (PIPLC). The GPI anchor targets PrP^C to caveolae-like domains (CLDs) (Gorodinsky and Harris 1995; Taraboulos et al. 1995; Vey et al. 1996; Naslavsky et al. 1997).

Formation of PrP^{Sc}

PrP^{Sc} accumulates in the brains of prion-infected animals while PrP mRNA levels remain unchanged (Oesch et al. 1985). These observations are consistent with metabolic labeling studies of prion-infected cultured cells, which have shown that PrP^C is synthesized and degraded rapidly whereas PrP^{Sc} is synthesized slowly by a posttranslational process (Borchelt et al. 1990; Caughey and Raymond 1991). Experimental results argue that PrP^C molecules exit to the cell surface prior to their conversion into PrP^{Sc} and only 10% of PrP^C molecules are then converted to PrP^{Sc}, presumably either in the endocytic pathway or on the plasma membrane (Caughey and Raymond 1991; Borchelt et al. 1992; Taraboulos et al. 1992b). Once PrP^{Sc} is formed, it is deposited in cytoplasmic vesicles, many of which appear to be secondary lysosomes (Borchelt et al. 1992; Taraboulos et al. 1990, 1992; McKinley et al. 1991; Caughey et al. 1991b).

The localization of PrP^C to CLDs and the finding that PrP^{Sc} formation is inhibited by lovastatin, which diminishes cellular cholesterol levels, suggested that glycosphingolipid- and cholesterol-rich CLDs might be the sites where prions are propagated (Taraboulos et al. 1995). Replacing the GPI anchor signal sequence with the CD4 transmembrane C-terminal 62 residues targeted the chimeric PrP molecule to clathrin-coated pits and prevented PrP^{Sc} formation. Furthermore, C-terminal truncation of PrP, which deleted the signal sequence for the GPI anchor, substantially reduced PrP^{Sc} formation (Rogers et al. 1993). Other studies have extended these observations by showing that squalestatin, a more specific inhibitor of cholesterol biosynthesis, and three other transmembrane C-terminal segments inhibit PrP^{Sc} formation (Kaneko et al. 1997a). Evidence exist that PrP^{Sc} interacts directly with PrP^C during the formation of nascent PrP^{Sc} (Prusiner et al. 1990; Telling et al. 1995; Horiuchi et al. 2000) and that this process occurs after PrP^C transits to the plasma membrane (Caughey and Raymond 1991; Borchelt et al. 1992). Our finding that antibody binding to cell-surface PrP^C alters PrP^{Sc} formation also supports this sequence of events (Peretz et al. 2001).

PrP^{Sc} can be labeled by the membrane-impermeable reagent sulfo-NHS-biotin when added to the growth medium of ScN2a cells, which indicates that some PrP^{Sc} is bound to the external surface of the plasma membrane. However, a substantial amount of PrP^{Sc} is found in lysosomes (Taraboulos et al. 1990; McKinley et al. 1991; Arnold et al. 1995). An auxiliary factor, provisionally designated protein X, has been implicated in the conversion of PrP^C into PrP^{Sc} based on the results of studies with transgenic mice (Telling et al. 1995). Additionally, the recognition site on PrP^C to which the putative protein X binds has been mapped using a series of chimeric PrP constructs expressed in ScN2a cells (Kaneko et al. 1997b).

Pathologic Changes in Prion Diseases and the Role of PrP^{Sc}

Pathologic changes in prion diseases include vacuolation of neurons and hypertrophy of astrocytes as well as the extracellular accumulation of PrP^{Sc} that polymerize to form amyloid fibrils. While the neuronal vacuolation and reactive astrocytic gliosis are generally obligatory characteristics of prion disease, PrP amyloid deposits are a variable feature (Prusiner et al. 1990).

The cell biology of PrP^{Sc} accumulation that leads to neuronal vacuolation remains unclear. Various studies argue that it is the intracellular accumulation of PrP^{Sc} that induces vacuolation of neurons (DeArmond et al. 1987). It has been suggested that, as neurons die, these vacuoles coalesce to form the spongy change seen in prion disease, with rare exception (DeArmond and Ironside 1999).

When primary cultures of neurons isolated from mouse brains were exposed to a PrP peptide corresponding to residues 100–126, the cells died (Forloni et al. 1993). However, when primary cultures of neurons isolated from brains of PrP-deficient ($Prnp^{0/0}$) mice were exposed to the same PrP peptide, the cells were unharmed (Brown et al. 1994). Consistent with these results are studies in which brain grafts were infected with prions and transplanted into the brains of $Prnp^{0/0}$ mice (Brandner et al. 1996). Although the cells of the graft produced large amounts of PrP^{Sc}, which were deposited extracellularly, the surrounding cells remained healthy. Taken together, these studies argue that the neurotoxicity of PrP^{Sc} is mediated through PrP^C.

BSE and variant CJD

In 1986, a previously unrecognized prion disease in cattle, termed bovine spongiform encephalopathy (BSE), was first identified in Great Britain (Wells et al. 1987). Investigations suggested that a dietary protein supplement, meat and bone meal (MBM), fed to cattle contained prions. Since scrapie, a prion disease in sheep, is endemic in Great Britain at high incidence, scrapie prions probably always have been present in slaughterhouse offal but were inactivated with organic solvents during the production of MBM. However, increased energy costs during the 1970s led to a decline in the use of these solvents in manufacturing MBM. It has been suggested that this change led to the contamination of MBM (Wilesmith et al. 1988). The incidence of infectivity probably increased dramatically when carcasses of cattle propagating BSE were used for MBM production, resulting in highly efficient intraspecies prion transmission. Another plausible explanation for the origin of the epidemic is that a spontaneous genetic mutation in cattle in the early 1980s created a bovine prion that contaminated MBM (Phillips et al. 2000). Unfortunately, the export of contaminated MBM from Great Britain led to the spread of BSE to other countries in Europe and possibly Asia.

In 1996, a new form of human prion disease, termed variant CJD (vCJD), was identified in the UK. vCJD displays a disease phenotype that is markedly different from previously known forms of CJD (Will et al. 1996; Ironside 1997). Many lines of research have supported epidemiological evidence implying that consumption of BSE-contaminated beef caused vCJD in humans (Lasmézas et al. 1996; Anderson et al. 1996; Collinge et al. 1996; Bruce et al. 1997; Hill et al. 1997; Wadsworth et al. 1999; Scott et al. 1999). More than 130 cases of vCJD have been reported to date. The suggestion that more than one million BSE-infected cattle were slaughtered for human consumption has fueled speculation that millions of consumers are at risk and has heightened the urgency for the development of effective therapeutics (Anderson et al. 1996).

PrP-Specific Antibodies

Prion infection fails to induce either the humoral or cellular response of the immune system. Given that PrP^C is expressed on the surface of many different tissues, it seems that mechanisms of immune tolerance prevent immune reactivity to it. More surprisingly, however, given the clear conformational differences observed between PrP^C and PrP^{Sc}, infected hosts appear to not view prion particles as foreign. Thus, immune tolerance restricts the anti-PrP antibody response to a small number of nonmurine PrP epitopes. An opportunity to access a wider spectrum of PrP-reactive monoclonal antibodies (mAbs) arose with the production of $Prnp^{0/0}$ mice (Büeler et al. 1992). Following immunization with PrP preparations, $Prnp^{0/0}$ mice produced antisera reacting strongly with PrP from several species, including mouse (Prusiner et al. 1993b).

PrP-specific mAbs recovered from immunized $Prnp^{0/0}$ mice were isolated via antigen-based selection from antibody fragment (Fab) libraries expressed on the surface of M13 phage. Fab libraries corresponding to four IgG isotypes, IgG1κ,

Table 1. Epitopes recognized and dissociation constants for the binding of PrP-specific Fabs to recombinant Syrian hamster PrP (29–231) refolded into an α-helical conformation. Binding constants were determined by surface plasmon resonance.

Fab	Epitope	K_d (μg/ml)	K_d (nM)
E123	29–37	3.45 ± 0.03	69 ± 0.5
E149	72–86	8.5 ± 0.03	170 ± 0.5
D13	95–103	0.16 ± 0.03	3.3 ± 0.5
D18	132–156	0.07 ± 0.03	1.6 ± 0.6
R72	151–162	No binding	No binding
R1	220–231	0.09 ± 0.04	1.7 ± 0.8
R2	225–231	0.11 ± 0.02	2.2 ± 0.5

IgG2aκ, IgG2bκ, and IgG3κ, were prepared from spleen, lymph node and bone marrow tissues taken from a mouse immunized with a variety of PrP isoforms (Williamson et al. 1996). Notably, only immunizations with PrP^{Sc} dispersed in liposomes yielded a large number of high affinity PrP-specific Fab clones, which reacted with human, bovine, sheep, Syrian hamster, and mouse PrP (Table 1) (Peretz et al. 1997; Williamson et al. 1998). Significantly, antibodies recognizing epitopes 90–120 bind PrP^{C} but not PrP^{Sc}, whereas antibodies recognizing residues 225–230 bound both isoforms, and antibodies recognizing residues 133--176 bound mostly PrP^{C} with some recognition of PrP^{Sc} (Peretz et al. 1997).

PrP-specific mAbs have also been raised in $Prnp^{0/0}$ mice, using traditional hybridoma fusion technology (Krasemann et al. 1996; Grassi et al. 2001). In one study, Korth et al. (1997) prepared hybridoma fusions from $Prnp^{0/0}$ mice immunized with recombinant bovine PrP. Two PrP-reactive mAbs were recovered: 6H4 recognized a single linear epitope of PrP between residues 144 and 152, and 15B3, of the IgM class was reported to recognize disease-specific forms of PrP, although later studies questioned this finding (Fischer et al. 2000).

Antibodies Bind Cell-Surface PrP^{C}

As direct interaction between PrP^{C} and PrP^{Sc} is proposed to drive the accumulation of nascent PrP^{Sc}, reagents specifically binding either PrP conformer may interrupt this pathological process. Antibodies to PrP are ideal candidates for such a therapeutic approach, as they have high affinities and are specific to PrP. The localization of PrP^{C} on the cell surface prior to its conversion into PrP^{Sc} makes it an easily accessible target for antibody binding.

To characterize plausible Fab–PrP interactions on the cell surface of ScN2a cells, we studied binding events with fluorescence-activated cell sorting (FACS). We found that antibodies bound PrP with different affinities and saturation levels. For example, D18 bound most of cell-surface PrP, D13 displayed higher affinities but bound less PrP at a saturation level, and R72 failed to bind PrP (Fig. 1b).

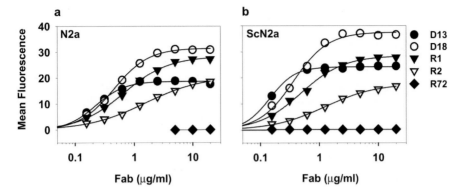

Fig. 1. PrP-specific antibody Fab binding to the surface of cells. The reactivities of PrP-specific Fabs D13, D18, R72, R1 and R2 with the surface of (**a**) N2a cells and (**b**) ScN2a cells were evaluated using flow cytometry. Panel **b** was reprinted with permission from Peretz et al. (2001).

To investigate which PrP isoform is bound, we measured Fab–PrP interactions on N2a cells that express only PrP^C (Fig. 1a). The formation characteristics of all Fab–PrP^C complexes were similar to those obtained with ScN2a cells (Fig. 1). Significantly, R1 and R2, which have been shown previously to bind both PrP^C and PrP^{Sc}, did not show higher binding signals with ScN2a cells. These similarities suggest that the main PrP isoform accessible to Fab binding on the surface of ScN2a cells is PrP^C.

Antibodies Inhibit PrP^{Sc} Formation in Cell Culture

Antibodies binding cell-surface PrP^C inhibited PrP^{Sc} formation in a dose-dependent manner. Fabs D13 and D18 appeared to be approximately equally effective, having IC_{50} values of 0.45 µg/ml (9 nM) and 0.6 µg/ml (12 nM), respectively. Fabs R1 and R2 were slightly less efficient, with IC_{50} values of 2.5 µg/ml (50 nM) and 2.0 µg/ml (40 nM), respectively. In contrast, Fabs E123, E149, R72, or 5-day treatment with polyclonal IgG, recognizing both transmembrane and GPI-anchored forms of mouse N-CAM, did not reduce the level of PrP^{Sc}, even when these antibodies were used at high concentrations (Fig. 2). The level of PrP^C in antibody-treated and untreated cells was found to be invariant, indicating that the PrP-specific antibodies did not alter the steady-state levels of PrP^C (Fig. 3).

When ScN2a cells were treated for two weeks with Fab D18, no PrP^{Sc} could be detected after four additional weeks of culture in antibody-free medium. Similarly, when ScN2a cells were treated with full length IgG mAb 6H4 for two consecutive weeks, followed by six weeks of growth in media without antibody, no PrP^{Sc} could be detected. Thus, transient treatment with PrP-specific antibodies led to the permanent elimination of PrP^{Sc} from cultured cells.

Elimination of PrP^{Sc} from ScN2a cells also diminished prion infectivity levels. Bioassays in which CD-1 Swiss mice were inoculated intracerebrally with lysates

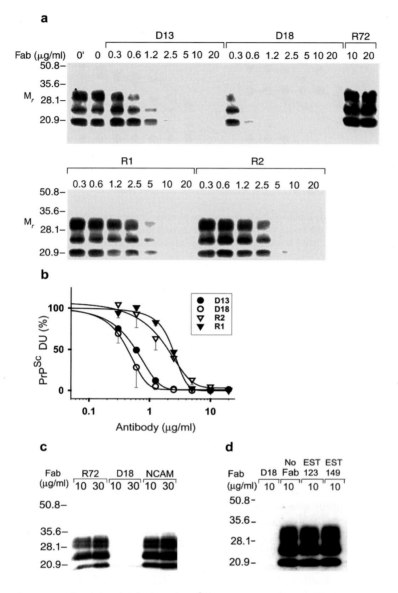

Fig. 2. Dose-dependent inhibition of PrP^{Sc} formation in ScN2a cell culture by PrP-specific recombinant antibody Fabs. (**a**) PrP^{Sc} levels in ScN2a cells were measured by immunoblotting following seven days of culture in the presence of antibodies D13, D18, R72, R1 or R2 at concentrations of 0–20 μg/ml. Lane 0' indicates the level of PrP^{Sc} in the ScN2a culture prior to antibody treatment. Protein sizes are shown as apparent molecular masses (M$_r$) in kDa. (**b**) Densitometric measurement of PrP^{Sc} bands identified in the immunoblot in panel **a**. Values are given as densitometric units (DU), where 100% is equivalent to the intensity of the PrP^{Sc} band in the absence of antibody treatment and 0% denotes undetectable levels of PrP^{Sc} in the culture (no band). Data represent the mean from three independent experiments. (**c**) PrP^{Sc} levels in ScN2a cells cultured for five days in the presence of anti-N-CAM polyclonal IgG, or (**d**) for seven days in the presence of Fabs E123 and E149. Reprinted with permission from Peretz et al.(2001).

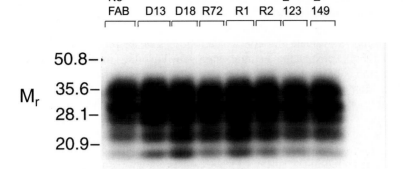

Fig. 3. Levels of PrP^C in antibody-treated ScN2a cells determined by immunoblot. ScN2a cultures were treated for a period of seven days with 10 μg/ml of Fabs D13, D18, R72, R1, R2, E123 or E149, or passaged in the absence of antibody. Reprinted with permission from Peretz et al. (2001).

Table 2. Bioassays of ScN2a cells treated with recombinant Fabs in CD-1 Swiss mice

Inoculum[a]	n/n_0[b]	Days ± SEM[c]
No Fab	9/9	169 ± 3
D13	0/10	>350
D18	0/8	>350
R72	10/10	165 ± 3
R1	9/10	206 ± 7
R2	0/7	>350

[a] Inoculum was a cell culture homogenate of ScN2a treated with antibodies.
[b] n, number of animals developing clinical signs of prion disease; n_0, total number of animals inoculated. Animals dying atypically following inoculation were excluded (Prusiner and McKinley 1987).
[c] Mean incubation period in days ± standard error of the mean (SEM).

of ScN2a cells treated for six weeks with various Fabs (D18, D13 or R2; 10 μg/ml) showed that the mice were disease-free after a period of more than 350 days. Mice inoculated with lysates of untreated or R72-treated cells had a mean incubation time to disease of 169 and 165 days, respectively (Table 2). The prolonged incubation times correspond to a reduction of over 3 logs in the infectious prion titer in treated cells. Consistent with the low inhibitory effect of R1 on PrP^{Sc} formation in cell culture, mice inoculated with R1-treated cells developed prion disease after 206 days. These data are consistent with the prion hypothesis, which proposes that the infectious prion particle is composed of PrP^{Sc}.

Transgenic Expression of Anti-PrP Antibodies in Mice Prevents Prion Disease

In studies aiming to evaluate the effect of antibodies on prion propagation in mice, Heppner et al. constructed a single chain gene encoding the epitope-binding variable regions of immunoglobulin heavy (VH) and light chains (VL) from cDNA of hybridoma cell lines 6H4 and 15B3 (Heppner et al. 2001). Expression of these sequences as transgenes in $Prnp^{0/0}$ mice resulted in sera with high titers of anti-PrP antibody in 6H4 but not 15B3. These transgenic (Tg) mice were bred with wild-type mice, resulting in $Prnp^{+/-}$-6H4 and $Prnp^{+/+}$-6H4 Tg lines. When Tg $Prnp^{+/-}$-6H4 mice were inoculated intraperitoneally with mouse prions, no infectivity could be detected in the spleen or CNS. Consistent with studies in cell culture, the transgenic expression of 6H4 did not affect steady-state levels of endogenous PrP^C in mice. The expression of 6H4 did not seem to induce symptoms of autoimmune disease in these mice.

Clearance of PrP^{Sc} from Cells Treated with Antibodies

A key question in therapeutic approaches to neurodegenerative diseases is the capacity of neurons to clear preexisting intracellular aggregates at the onset of the treatment. The data presented might be taken to indicate that PrP^{Sc} levels rapidly diminish (Fig. 1). Indeed, data reported in other studies describing the inhibition of prion propagation have been interpreted in this way. However, these studies did not take the mitotic expansion of cells in culture into consideration. To measure the rate at which PrP^{Sc} is eliminated from cultures, one must account for the increase in cell population and the commensurate reduction in PrP^{Sc} concentration that take place over the course of the experiment.

To analyze the kinetics of prion clearance, cells were independently grown in the presence of PrP-specific Fabs and harvested after a period of 1, 2, 3, and 4 days of antibody treatment, and the total mass of protein was determined in each case as a measure of cell number (Fig. 4). Total PrP^{Sc} in the culture at each time point, determined by immunoblotting, was then calculated by factoring in the total cell mass in each case. In agreement with earlier results, Fab D18 was found to be the most effective antibody. The time elapsed from initial treatment with D18 to elimination of 50% of PrP^{Sc} from cells ($t_{1/2}$) was 28 hours (Table 3). The $t_{1/2}$ of PrP^{Sc} in ScN2a cells is thought to exceed 24 hours, suggesting that, at a concentration of 10 µg/ml, Fab D18 is able to completely abolish prion propagation and that pre-existing PrP^{Sc} is subsequently eliminated. This finding indicates that a certain amount of PrP^{Sc} is continuously removed from ScN2a cultures through degradation pathways. Fab D13 was the next most potent antibody, also lowering the level of PrP^{Sc}, but to a lesser extent than Fab D18, indicating that there may be a minimal level of residual PrP^{Sc} synthesis in the presence of this Fab. Fabs R1 and R2, although clearly reducing the rate of prion propagation in ScN2a cells, are not sufficiently effective to yield a reduction in the overall quantity of PrP^{Sc} present in the culture. In untreated cultures, or cultures treated with Fab R72, prion propagation remained unaffected, and PrP^{Sc} levels increased in tandem with a growth in the ScN2a cell population.

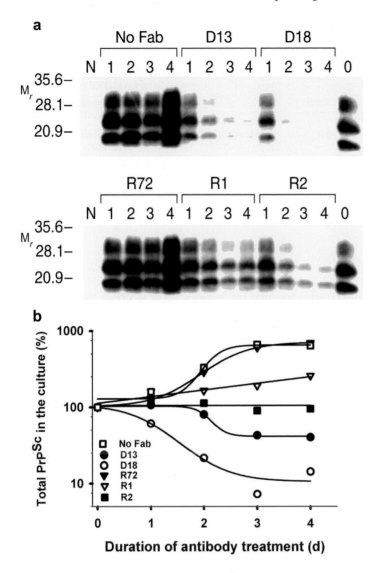

Fig. 4. Time course of antibody-mediated PrP^Sc clearance. (**a**) The level of PrP^Sc in ScN2a cells grown for 1, 2, 3 or 4 days in the presence of PrP-specific Fabs (10 μg/ml) was determined by immunoblotting. (**b**) The effect of antibody treatment on the total amount of PrP^Sc in ScN2a cell cultures. Lane N indicates N2a cells treated with proteinase K. The data represent the mean of three experiments. Reprinted with permission from Peretz et al. (2001).

Table 3. Summary of $t_{1/2}$ values for PrP synthesis and degradation in N2a and ScN2a cells.

Parameter measured	N2a	ScN2a	Method and reference
Synthesis of PrP^C	< 2.5 min	< 2.5 min	Metabolic radiolabeling, (Borchelt et al. 1992)
Synthesis[a] of PrP^{Sc}	None	3 h	Metabolic radiolabeling, (Borchelt et al. 1990)
Degradation of PrP^C	6 h	Undetermined	Metabolic radiolabeling, (Borchelt et al. 1990)
Degradation[b] of PrP^{Sc}	None	28 h	Fab inhibition, (Peretz et al. 2001)

[a] Refers to the acquisition of protease-resistant PrP.
[b] Refers to the elimination of protease-resistant PrP.

Conclusions

The present findings clearly show that antibodies specific to PrP can inhibit prion formation in infected cell cultures. It is also clear that the efficiency of this process varies dramatically between individual antibodies. Mechanistically, the inhibitory effect is most readily explained by antibody binding specifically to PrP^C molecules on the cell surface and thereby impeding binding to the PrP^{Sc} template or another cofactor critical for prion formation. In agreement with this hypothesis, Fab D18, which was by far the most effective antibody evaluated, was distinguished by its capacity to bind a significantly greater number of cell-surface PrP^C molecules than other Fabs. We conclude that the amount of cell-surface PrP^C occupied by a given antibody is a key determinant of the inhibitory potency of that antibody.

In addition to cell-surface PrP^C binding, the inhibitory potency of each Fab depends upon the region of PrP it binds. For example, at concentrations of 0.6 μg/ml and 2.5 μg/ml, respectively, Fabs D18 and R1 bound equivalently to ScN2a cells, but D18 was clearly more effective in reducing the level of PrP^{Sc} in culture. Similarly, at a concentration of 2.5 μg/ml, Fabs D13 and R1 bound equivalently to the cell surface, but D13 more actively reduced PrP^{Sc} synthesis. Numerous reports identify the binding site of D18 (residues 132–156) as critical for efficient interspecies transmission of prions; we therefore argue that D18 operates by directly blocking PrP^C interaction with PrP^{Sc} (Scott et al. 1993; Kocisko et al. 1995; Priola and Chesebro 1995; Priola et al. 2001). Thus, the potent activity of Fab D18 is associated with its ability to recognize better the total population of PrP^C on the cell surface and with the location of its epitope on PrP^C.

The mechanism implicated in antibody inhibition of prion formation seems to differ from those suggested by studies with amyloid precursor protein (APP) in a transgenic mouse model of Alzheimer's disease. Immunization of APP transgenic mice with Aβ peptide led to antibody formation and subsequent reduction of amyloid deposits in the CNS (Schenk et al. 1999). This event seems to be mediated, in part, through plaque-binding antibodies that trigger Fc-mediated phagocytosis of Aβ by microglia cells (Bard et al. 2000). It was also suggested that Aβ is in equilibrium between the CNS and the plasma and that the formation of antibody-Aβ in the plasma alters this equilibrium to result in increased Aβ serum levels, which subsequently leads to decreased Aβ deposits in the brain (DeMattos et al. 2001, 2002). Another plausible mechanism arises from the demonstration that antibodies specific to Aβ modulate its solubility and aggregation *in vitro* (Frenkel et al. 1999).

Studies with PrP propose another plausible mechanism for antibody-mediated inhibition of protein deposition (Peretz et al. 2001). Antibodies binding to specific key epitopes of a protein destined for amyloid formation could result in complexes inherent for aggregation and therefore might be used as therapeutic reagents for diseases caused by protein deposition.

In summary, it has been shown that antibodies binding to defined regions of PrP^C effectively inhibit prion replication in cell culture. For *in vivo* applications, Fabs have the disadvantage of a short half-life. Humanized whole antibody molecules prepared from Fabs or from hybridoma-derived IgG antibodies will likely be more useful, but may require engineering to prevent the recruitment of immunologic effector mechanisms to antibody-coated cells. The studies described here, in combination with recent advances targeting Alzheimer's disease, indicate that specific antibodies may become powerful weapons in the fight against neurodegenerative diseases associated with the accumulation of misfolded proteins.

References

Anderson RM, Donnelly CA, Ferguson NM, Woolhouse ME, Watt CJ, Udy HJ, MaWhinney S, Dunstan SP, Southwood TR, Wilesmith JW, Ryan JB, Hoinville LJ, Hillerton JE, Austin AR, Wells GA (1996) Transmission dynamics and epidemiology of BSE in British cattle. Nature 382:779–788

Arnold JE, Tipler C, Laszlo L, Hope J, Landon M, Mayer RJ (1995) The abnormal isoform of the prion protein accumulates in late-endosome-like organelles in scrapie-infected mouse brain. J Pathol 176:403–411

Bard F, Cannon C, Barbour R, Burke RL, Games D, Grajeda H, Guido T, Hu K, Huang J, Johnson-Wood K, Khan K, Kholodenko D, Lee M, Lieberburg I, Motter R, Nguyen M, Soriano F, Vasquez N, Weiss K, Welch B, Seubert P, Schenk D, Yednock T (2000) Peripherally administered antibodies against amyloid β-peptide enter the central nervous system and reduce pathology in a mouse model of Alzheimer disease. Nature Med 6:916–919

Basler K, Oesch B, Scott M, Westaway D, Walchli M, Groth DF, McKinley MP, Prusiner SB, Weissmann C (1986) Scrapie and cellular PrP isoforms are encoded by the same chromosomal gene. Cell 46:417–428

Borchelt DR, Scott M, Taraboulos A, Stahl N, Prusiner SB (1990) Scrapie and cellular prion proteins differ in their kinetics of synthesis and topology in cultured cells. J Cell Biol 110:743–752

Borchelt DR, Taraboulos A, Prusiner SB (1992) Evidence for synthesis of scrapie prion proteins in the endocytic pathway. J Biol Chem 267:16188–16199

Brandner S, Isenmann S, Raeber A, Fischer M, Sailer A, Kobayashi Y, Marino S, Weissmann C, Aguzzi A (1996) Normal host prion protein necessary for scrapie-induced neurotoxicity. Nature 379:339–343

Brown DR, Herms J, Kretzschmar HA (1994) Mouse cortical cells lacking cellular PrP survive in culture with a neurotoxic PrP fragment. Neuroreport 5:2057–2060

Bruce ME, Will RG, Ironside JW, McConnell I, Drummond D, Suttie A, McCardle L, Chree A, Hope J, Birkett C, Cousens S, Fraser H, Bostock CJ (1997) Transmissions to mice indicate that 'new variant' CJD is caused by the BSE agent. Nature 389:498–501

Bueler H, Fischer M, Lang Y, Bluethmann H, Lipp HP, DeArmond SJ, Prusiner SB, Aguet M, Weissmann C (1992) Normal development and behaviour of mice lacking the neuronal cell-surface PrP protein. Nature 356:577–582

Caughey B, Raymond GJ (1991) The scrapie-associated form of PrP is made from a cell surface precursor that is both protease- and phospholipase-sensitive. J Biol Chem 266:18217–18223

Caughey B, Raymond GJ, Ernst D, Race RE (1991b) N-terminal truncation of the scrapie-associated form of PrP by lysosomal protease(s): implications regarding the site of conversion of PrP to the protease-resistant state. J Virol 65:6597–6603

Caughey BW, Dong A, Bhat KS, Ernst D, Hayes SF, Caughey WS (1991a) Secondary structure analysis of the scrapie-associated protein PrP 27-30 in water by infrared spectroscopy. Biochemistry 30:7672–7680

Cohen FE, Prusiner SB (1998) Pathologic conformations of prion proteins. Annu Rev Biochem 67:793–819

Collinge J, Sidle KCL, Meads J, Ironside J, Hill AF (1996) Molecular analysis of prion strain variation and the aetiology of "new variant" CJD. Nature 383:685–690

DeArmond SJ, Ironside JW (1999) Neuropathology of prion disease. In: Prusiner SB (ed) *Prion biology and diseases.* Cold Spring Harbor Laboratory Press, Cold Spring Harbor, pp. 585–652

DeArmond SJ, Mobley WC, DeMott DL, Barry RA, Beckstead JH, Prusiner SB (1987) Changes in the localization of brain prion proteins during scrapie infection. Neurology 37:1271–1280

DeMattos RB, Bales KR, Cummins DJ, Dodart JC, Paul SM, Holtzman DM (2001) Peripheral anti-A beta antibody alters CNS and plasma A beta clearance and decreases brain A beta burden in a mouse model of Alzheimer's disease. Proc Natl Acad Sci USA 98:8850–8855

DeMattos RB, Bales KR, Cummins,DJ, Paul SM, Holtzman DM (2002) Brain to plasma amyloid-beta efflux: a measure of brain amyloid burden in a mouse model of Alzheimer's disease. Science 295:2264–2267

Enari M, Flechsig E, &Weissmann C (2001) Scrapie prion protein accumulation by scrapie-infected neuroblastoma cells abrogated by exposure to a prion protein antibody. Proc Natl Acad Sci USA 98:9295–9299

Fischer MB, Roeckl C, Parizek P, Schwarz HP, Aguzzi A (2000) Binding of disease-associated prion protein to plasminogen. Nature 408:479–483

Forloni G, Angeretti N, Chiesa R, Monzani E, Salmona M, Bugiani O, Tagliavini F (1993) Neurotoxicity of a prion protein fragment. Nature 362:543–546

Frenkel D, Balass M, Katchalski-Katzir E, Solomon B (1999) High affinity binding of monoclonal antibodies to the sequential epitope EFRH of beta-amyloid peptide is essential for modulation of fibrillar aggregation. J Neuroimmunol 95:136–142

Gasset M, Baldwin MA, Fletterick RJ, Prusiner SB (1993) Perturbation of the secondary structure of the scrapie prion protein under conditions that alter infectivity. Proc Natl Acad Sci USA 90:1–5

Gorodinsky A, Harris DA (1995) Glycolipid-anchored proteins in neuroblastoma cells form detergent-resistant complexes without caveolin. J Cell Biol 129:619–627

Grassi J, Comoy E, Simon S, Creminon C, Frobert Y, Trapmann S, Schimmel H, Hawkins SA, Moynagh J, Deslys JP, Wells GA (2001) Rapid test for the preclinical postmortem diagnosis of BSE in central nervous system tissue. Vet Rec 149:577–582

Heppner FL, Musahl C, Arrighi I, Klein MA, Rulicke T, Oesch B, Zinkernagel RM, Kalinke U, Aguzzi A (2001) Prevention of scrapie pathogenesis by transgenic expression of anti-prion protein antibodies. Science 294:178–182

Hill AF, Desbruslais M, Joiner S, Sidle KC, Gowland I, Collinge J, Doey LJ, Lantos P (1997) The same prion strain causes vCJD and BSE. Nature 389:448–450

Hope J, Morton LJ, Farquhar CF, Multhaup G, Beyreuther K, Kimberlin RH (1986) The major polypeptide of scrapie-associated fibrils (SAF) has the same size, charge distribution and N-terminal protein sequence as predicted for the normal brain protein (PrP). EMBO J 5:2591–2597

Horiuchi M, Chabry J, Caughey B (1999) Specific binding of normal prion protein to the scrapie form via a localized domain initiates its conversion to the protease-resistant state. EMBO J 18:3193–3203

Horiuchi M, Priola SA, Chabry J, Caughey B (2000) Interactions between heterologous forms of prion protein: binding, inhibition of conversion, and species barriers. Proc Natl Acad Sci USA 97:5836–5841

Ironside JW (1997) The new variant form of Creutzfeldt-Jakob disease: a novel prion protein amyloid disorder (Editorial). Amyloid 4:66–69

Kaneko K, Vey M, Scott M, Pilkuhn S, Cohen FE, Prusiner SB (1997a) COOH-terminal sequence of the cellular prion protein directs subcellular trafficking and controls conversion into the scrapie isoform. Proc Natl Acad Sci USA 94:2333–2338

Kaneko K, Zulianello L, Scott M, Cooper CM, Wallace AC, James TL, Cohen FE, Prusiner SB (1997b) Evidence for protein X binding to a discontinuous epitope on the cellular prion protein during scrapie prion propagation. Proc Natl Acad Sci USA 94:10069–10074

Kaytor MD, Warren ST (1999) Aberrant protein deposition and nevrological disease. J Biol Chem 274:37507–37510

Kitamoto T, Ogomori K, Tateishi J, Prusiner SB (1987) Formic acid pretreatment enhances immunostaining of cerebral and systemic amyloids. Lab Invest 57:230–236

Kocisko DA, Priola SA, Raymond GJ, Chesebro B, Lansbury PT Jr, Caughey B (1995) Species specificity in the cell-free conversion of prion protein to protease-resistant forms: a model for the scrapie species barrier. Proc Natl Acad Sci USA 92:3923–3927

Korth C, Stierli B, Streit P, Moser M, Schaller O, Fischer R, Schulz-Schaeffer W, Kretzschmar H, Raeber A, Braun U, Ehrensperger F, Hornemann S, Glockshuber R, Riek R, Billeter M, Wuthrich K, Oesch B (1997) Prion (PrP^{Sc})-specific epitope defined by a monoclonal antibody. Nature 389:74–77

Krasemann S, Groschup M, Hunsmann G. Bodemer W (1996) Induction of antibodies against human prion proteins (PrP) by DNA-mediated immunization of PrP$^{0/0}$ mice. J Immunol Methods 199:109–118

Lasmezas CI, Deslys JP, Demaimay R, Adjou KT, Lamoury F, Dormont D, Robain O, Ironside J, Hauw JJ (1996) BSE transmission to macaques. Nature 381:743–744

McKinley MP, Taraboulos A, Kenaga L, Serban D, Stieber A, DeArmond SJ, Prusiner SB, Gonatas N (1991) Ultrastructural localization of scrapie prion proteins in cytoplasmic vesicles of infected cultured cells. Lab Invest 65:622–630

Naslavsky N, Stein R, Yanai A, Friedlander G, Taraboulos A (1997) Characterization of detergent-insoluble complexes containing the cellular prion protein and its scrapie isoform. J Biol Chem 272:6324–6331

Oesch B, Jensen M, Nilsson P, Fogh J (1994) Properties of the scrapie prion protein: Quantitative analysis of protease resistance. Biochemistry 33:5926–5931

Oesch B, Westaway D, Walchli M, McKinley MP, Kent SB, Aebersold R, Barry RA, Tempst P, Teplow DB, Hood LE (1985) A cellular gene encodes scrapie PrP 27-30 protein. Cell 40:735–746

Pan KM, Baldwin M, Nguyen J, Gasset M, Serban A, Groth D, Mehlhorn I, Huang Z, Fletterick RJ, Cohen FE, Prusiner SB (1993) Conversion of α-helices into β-sheets features in the formation of the scrapie prion proteins. Proc Natl Acad Sci USA 90:10962–10966

Peretz D, Williamson RA, Kaneko K, Vergara J, Leclerc E, Schmitt-Ulms G, Mehlhorn IR, Legname G, Wormald MR, Rudd PM, Dwek RA, Burton DR, Prusiner SB (2001) Antibodies inhibit prion propagation and clear cell cultures of prion infectivity. Nature 412:739–743

Peretz D, Williamson RA, Legname G, Matsunaga Y, Vergara J, Burton DR, DeArmond SJ, Prusiner SB, Scott MR (2002) A change in the conformation of prions accompanies the emergence of a new prion strain. Neuron 34:921–932

Peretz D, Williamson RA, Matsunaga Y, Serban H, Pinilla C, Bastidas RB, Rozenshteyn R, James TL, Houghten RA, Cohen FE, Prusiner SB, Burton DR (1997) A conformational transition at the N-terminus of the prion protein features in formation of the scrapie isoform. J Mol Biol 273:614–622

Pergami P, Jaffe H, Safar J (1996) Semipreparative chromatographic method to purify the normal cellular isoform of the prion protein in nondenatured form. Anal Biochem 236:63–73

Phillips NA, Bridgeman J, Ferguson-Smith M (2000) In: The BSE Inquiry Report October 24, Stationery Office, London

Priola SA, Chabry J, Chan K (2001) Efficient conversion of normal prion protein (PrP) by abnormal hamster PrP is determined by homology at amino acid residue 155. J Virol 75:4673–4680

Priola SA, Chesebro B (1995) A single hamster PrP amino acid blocks conversion to protease-resistant PrP in scrapie-infected mouse neuroblastoma cells. J Virol 69:7754–7758

Prusiner SB (1998) Prions. Proc Natl Acad Sci USA 95:13363–13383

Prusiner SB Groth DF, Bolton DC, Kent SB, Hood LE (1984) Purification and structural studies of a major scrapie prion protein. Cell 38:127–134

Prusiner SB, Groth D, Serban A, Koehler R, Foster D, Torchia M, Burton D, Yang SL, DeArmond SJ (1993b) Ablation of the prion protein (PrP) gene in mice prevents scrapie and facilitates production of anti-PrP antibodies. Proc Natl Acad Sci USA 90:10608–10612

Prusiner SB, Groth D, Serban A, Stahl N, Gabizon R (1993a) Attempts to restore scrapie prion infectivity after exposure to protein denaturants. Proc Natl Acad Sci USA 90:2793–2797

Prusiner SB, McKinley MP, Bowman KA, Bolton DC, Bendheim PE, Groth DF, Glenner GG (1983) Scrapie prions aggregate to form amyloid-like birefringent rods. Cell 35:349–358

Prusiner SB, Scott M, Foster D, Pan KM, Groth D, Mirenda C, Torchia M, Yang SL, Serban D, Carlson GA (1990) Transgenetic studies implicate interactions between homologous PrP isoforms in scrapie prion replication. Cell 63:673–686

Rogers M, Yehiely F, Scott M, Prusiner SB (1993) Conversion of truncated and elongated prion proteins into the scrapie isoform in cultured cells. Proc Natl Acad Sci USA 90:3182–3186

Safar J, Roller PP, Gajdusek DC, Gibbs CJJ (1993) Thermal-stability and conformational transitions of scrapie amyloid (prion) protein correlate with infectivity. Protein Sci 2:2206–2216

Schenk D, Barbour R, Dunn W, Gordon G, Grajeda H, Guido T, Hu K, Huang J, Johnson-Wood K, Khan K, Kholodenko D, Lee M, Liao Z, Lieberburg I, Motter R, Mutter L, Soriano F, Shopp G, Vasquez N, Vandevert C, Walker S, Wogulis M, Yednock T, Games D, Seubert P (1999) Immunization with amyloid-beta attenuates Alzheimer-disease-like pathology in the PDAPP mouse. Nature 400:173–177

Scott M, Foster D, Mirenda C, Serban D, Coufal F, Walchli M, Torchia M, Groth D, Carlson G, DeArmond SJ (1989) Transgenic mice expressing hamster prion protein produce species-specific scrapie infectivity and amyloid plaques. Cell 59:847–857

Scott M, Groth D, Foster D, Torchia M, Yang SL, DeArmond SJ, Prusiner SB (1993) Propagation of prions with artificial properties in transgenic mice expressing chimeric PrP genes. Cell 73:979–988

Scott MR, Will R, Ironside J, Nguyen HO, Tremblay P, DeArmond SJ, Prusiner SB (1999) Compelling transgenetic evidence for transmission of bovine spongiform encephalopathy prions to humans. Proc Natl Acad Sci USA 96:15137–15142

Serban D, Taraboulos A, DeArmond SJ, Prusiner SB (1990) Rapid detection of Creutzfeldt-Jakob disease and scrapie prion proteins. Neurology 40:110–117

Stahl N, Baldwin MA, Burlingame AL, Prusiner SB (1990) Identification of glycoinositol phospholipid linked and truncated forms of the scrapie prion protein. Biochemistry 29:8879–8884

Stahl N, Baldwin MA, Hecker R, Pan KM, Burlingame AL, Prusiner SB (1992) Glycosylinositol phospholipid anchors of the scrapie and cellular prion proteins contain sialic acid. Biochemistry 31:5043–5053

Stahl N, Borchelt DR, Hsiao K, Prusiner SB (1987) Scrapie prion protein contains a phosphatidylinositol glycolipid. Cell 51:229–240

Taraboulos A, Jendroska K, Serban D, Yang SL, DeArmond SJ, Prusiner SB (1992a) Regional mapping of prion proteins in brains. Proc Natl Acad Sci USA 89:7620–7624

Taraboulos A, Raeber AJ, Borchelt DR, Serban D, Prusiner SB (1992b) Synthesis and trafficking of prion proteins in cultured cells. Mol Biol Cell 3:851–863

Taraboulos A, Scott M, Semenov A, Laszlo L, Prusiner SB, Avraham D (1995) Cholesterol depletion and modification of COOH-terminal targeting sequence of the prion protein inhibits formation of the scrapie isoform. J Cell Biol 129:121–132

Taraboulos A, Serban D, Prusiner SB (1990) Scrapie prion proteins accumulate in the cytoplasm of persistently infected cultured cells. J Cell Biol 110:2117–2132

Telling GC, Parchi P, DeArmond SJ, Cortelli P, Montagna P, Gabizon R, Mastrianni J, Lugaresi E, Gambetti P, Prusiner SB (1996) Evidence for the conformation of the pathologic isoform of the prion protein enciphering and propagating prion diversity. Science 274:2079–2082

Telling GC, Scott M, Mastrianni J, Gabizon R, Torchia M, Cohen FE, DeArmond SJ, Prusiner SB (1995) Prion propagation in mice expressing human and chimeric PrP transgenes implicates the interaction of cellular PrP with another protein. Cell 83:79–90

Turk E, Teplow DB, Hood LE, Prusiner SB (1988) Purification and properties of the cellular and scrapie hamster prion proteins. Eur J Biochem 176:21–30

Vey M, Pilkuhn S, Wille H, Nixon R, DeArmond SJ, Smart EJ, Anderson RG, Taraboulos A, Prusiner SB (1996) Subcellular colocalization of the cellular and scrapie prion proteins in caveolae-like membranous domains. Proc Natl Acad Sci USA 93:14945–14949

Wadsworth JD, Hill AF, Joiner S, Jackson GS, Clarke AR, Collinge J (1999) Strain-specific prion-protein conformation determined by metal ions. Nature Cell Biol 1:55–59

Wells GA, Scott AC, Johnson CT, Gunning RF, Hancock RD, Jeffrey M, Dawson M, Bradley R (1987) A novel progressive spongiform encephalopathy in cattle. Vet Rec 121:419–420

Wilesmith JW, Wells GAH, Cranwell MP, Ryan JBM (1988) Bovine spongiform encephalopathy: epidemiological studies. Vet Rec 123:638–644

Will RG, Alpers MP, Dormont D, Schonberger LB, Tateishi J (1999) Infectious and sporadic prion diseases In: Prusiner SB (ed) Prion biology and diseases. Cold Spring Harbor Laboratory Press, Cold Spring Harbor, pp. 465–507

Will RG, Ironside JW, Zeidler M, Cousens SN, Estibeiro K, Alperovitch A, Poser S, Pocchiari M, Hofman A, Smith PG (1996) A new variant of Creutzfeldt-Jakob disease in the UK. Lancet 347:921–925

Williamson RA, Peretz D, Pinilla C, Ball H, Bastidas RB, Rozenshteyn R, Houghten RA, Prusiner SB, Burton DR (1998) Mapping the prion protein using recombinant antibodies. J Virol 72:9413–9418

Williamson RA, Peretz D, Smorodinsky N, Bastidas R, Serban H, Mehlhorn I, DeArmond SJ, Prusiner SB, Burton DR (1996) Circumventing tolerance to generate autologous monoclonal antibodies to the prion protein. Proc Natl Acad Sci USA 93:7279–7282

Prusiner SB, McKinley MP(1987) (eds) Prions: novel infectious pathogens causing scrapie and Creutzfeldt-Jakob disease. Academic Press, Orlando .

Subject Index

Printing: Saladruck Berlin
Binding: Stürtz AG, Würzburg